Becoming the Next
BABY SLEEP BOSS

Teaching Your Baby
How to *Thrive* Through the Day
and *Sleep* Through the Night

Taylor Fontenot, RN, BSN

kindle direct publishing

Legal Disclaimer:

This book contains information that parents can use as a guide for their baby's first year of life. Please note that you should always consult your pediatrician when making decisions regarding your baby's health, behavior, and sleep routines. This information is designed for healthy, full-term babies and is not intended to replace medical advice.

ISBN 978-0-578-55536-2

Front cover and back cover baby photo (my darling niece) © 2018 Caroline Fontenot

Author photo © 2019 Lindsey Locker

First Edition

*This book is dedicated to tired
parents across the globe.*

*May this information
provide you with an extra
dose of the sleep and sanity
you deserve.*

CONTENTS

Imagine living out motherhood from now until forever, without guilt. Imagine caring for your children and yourself simultaneously without constantly questioning every decision you make. It's possible. It's also a choice.

- Rachel Hollis, *Girl, Wash Your Face*

No discipline seems pleasant at the time, but painful. Later on, however, it produces a harvest of righteousness and peace by those who have been trained by it.

- The Apostle Paul, *Hebrews 12:11*

Sleep deprivation is not so bad.

- No one, ever

INTRODUCTION

Hi, I'm Taylor...

Part-time nurse, full-time boy mom, lover of sleep.

When I had my first baby in 2014, I was consumed by all the resources provided for life leading up to birth – 6-week labor courses, doula contacts, hypnobirthing, you name it – but I couldn't believe how little was said about *after* the baby is born. Being the learner that I am, I knew I needed a plan. I had seen too many friends try to "wing it" and end up merely surviving their first year of parenthood, hardly enjoying or even remembering it. Maybe you can relate!

I combed through all the baby books I could find and landed on some parenting approaches that made sense to me. However, I consistently ran into two main issues: 1) The book layouts were confusing and wordy, and 2) The lingo was incredibly dry and boring. I wanted to be able to teach my baby how to sleep through the night; I wanted to raise a strong, independent child; I wanted to maintain some structure in my home and, more importantly, my marriage, but I longed for it to come from a resource that provided the right information while also empathizing with all the varying emotions I experienced through motherhood. I didn't want stern advice from a 60-something guy with a PhD; I wanted light-hearted, real lingo from a mom who had walked in my shoes and understood my parenting anxieties. I never found that resource, so I decided to write it myself!

This book is a compilation of sleep strategies and baby basics obtained from multiple resources but tweaked to fit the modern family. My husband and I trialed these concepts with our first baby and were beyond thrilled when our transition to parenthood went smoothly AND our baby started sleeping through the night at just eight weeks of age. The strategies had worked, but I still wasn't convinced. Maybe we were just lucky. Certainly, some babies are born with "easier" demeanors than others. After raising two more babies (with very different personalities) using this method and finding that all three were miracle sleepers, I became a believer!

When I tell people that I have three boys (all two years apart), the comments regarding sleep are endless: "Oh wow, you've got your hands full! I guess you'll sleep in your next life!" I always chuckle to myself because my boys are currently one, three and five years old and – between you and me – I sleep eight solid hours a night. Seriously. I have always needed this much sleep, I feared that motherhood would take that away, and I'm here to tell you that it doesn't have to.

Attaining this kind of rest with a house full of littles does not come by coincidence. For this reason – using the mind of a nurse and the heart of a mom – I created "The Baby Sleep Boss (BSB) Method." Now I am passionate about sharing this method with others and coaching them through these first twelve months that, I believe, can make or break your opinion of parenthood and your enjoyment of life. This is no small deal, y'all! I want everyone to love and cherish this first year as much as I have. I want everyone to go into subsequent babies with joy and anticipation rather than fear and dread. I want everyone to experience order in their homes and long nights of sleep. I want marriages and partnerships to THRIVE, not just survive.

My Beliefs on Parenting

To help you understand how I developed this method and whether or not this may be right for your family, let's start with some of my beliefs on parenting. First and foremost, I believe that a baby is to be welcomed into *your* world and thus adjust to fit it accordingly. I believe that a strong partnership between a mom and dad is the hallmark to successful parenting and that the love you have for your child comes second to this relationship. I still believe in prioritizing my husband, dating him, and spending quality time with him doing activities we both enjoy. Because we have set this precedence over our household, our children know that our relationship is of the utmost importance and I truly believe they feel secure and loved because of that. When my husband and I have a date night, our boys celebrate it, ask us where we're going, and can't wait to hear about it. We feel confident about leaving them with a babysitter because they have a simple bedtime routine that can be implemented by anyone. They are secure in our love for them because we are modeling that toward each other first.

I also want to acknowledge that this mom-dad parenting relationship is not a reality for everyone. There is much to benefit from this book no matter what type of family you inhabit, but for simplicity's sake, my lingo will be addressing a man and woman parenthood partnership. Single parents, stay-at-home dads, adoptive parents and LGBTQ partnerships, I welcome you and hope you will feel included and encouraged through this journey as well.

Note: As a mom of three boys, it comes naturally to address a baby using masculine pronouns, so I will do this as a means of consistency throughout the text, even though I love me some girl babies too!

What is The Baby Sleep Boss (BSB) Method?

The BSB Method is a structured approach to "gradual sleep training" with goals to maintain sanity in your home and long nights of sleep for the entire family. With this method you will learn how to teach your baby self-soothing techniques so that he can fall asleep independently. The belief is that, by providing small adjustments in your baby's habits from day one, he can gently and gradually learn how to develop a daily nap routine and sleep through the night.

One of the most important concepts of The BSB Method is learning how to put your baby down to sleep while he is drowsy but still awake. I like to call this "staying ahead of the meltdown." Let me explain. In my role as a Registered Nurse, I am continually assessing my patients for signs and symptoms of pain and intervening as soon as possible to prevent the pain from getting worse. In the nursing world, we call this "staying ahead of the pain." The goal is to treat the pain before it gets out of hand so that we aren't having to play catch-up. In my role as a mom, I have found that the exact same method can be applied to our babies and their sleep. If we learn how to watch our babies and recognize signs and symptoms of *drowsiness*, we can put them down to sleep *before* the meltdown occurs. In the same way that we are not letting pain get out of control, we are not letting our baby's exhaustion get out of control. This is a vital concept of sleep training that I'll discuss more in Chapter 4 (Week Two).

Why is sleep training a baby so important in the first place? Because sleep deprivation can wreak havoc on the health of your whole family. Let's take a moment to reflect back on the way you felt the morning after you pulled that all-nighter in college. You may remember feeling fatigue, fogginess, irritability, or hardly remember it at all. Now do that every night for the next year (or more) of your life and just imagine how crazy you could become! Lack of sleep makes it more difficult for us to solve problems, juggle multiple tasks, understand the perspectives of others, and regulate our emotions.[1] It can lead to dangerous feelings of disappointment or even anger toward your child.[2] Additionally, babies who have poor sleeping habits have a higher incidence of daytime fussiness, colic-like symptoms, poor eating habits, and learning and behavioral deficiencies, such as ADHD.[3] Sound like a fun home environment? Yikes! I'm not trying to scare you; I'm trying to *prepare* you. No first-time parent can fully understand the horrors of sleep deprivation until they are in it, but my hope is that I can equip you with skills that will prevent this from becoming your reality in the first place. I truly believe that one of our greatest roles as parents is to educate ourselves so that we can gently and adequately teach our children how to sleep.

Does this have to be militant? Absolutely not! The goal is to provide your baby with a consistent routine so that he can be flexible. *How does this make sense?* Because when you are in charge and you repeatedly give your baby a reliable structure he can depend on, he will trust you. He will know that you continually provide what he needs, and he can stop trying to be the boss. We live in a world that is notorious for raising selfish, entitled human beings that require instant gratification. Call me crazy, but I truly believe this starts at the beginning. This is not just a small issue of sleep but a concept that envelops your entire approach to parenting. Do you want a household run by your child? Do you think it's cute to be wrapped around Little Johnny's finger? This happens more easily than you would think! Instead, by setting a precedence early, we can teach our children that we, as their parents, actually know what is best for them. We can utilize our knowledge and confidence in regard to sleep, and this authority will trickle down into all other facets of parenting. This is beneficial to the entire family.

All that to say, The BSB Method is not for everyone. I am organized, a tiny bit type-A, and love structure in my life, so having a plan and a system fits my personality. It also takes some work and conscious effort up-front and therefore may feel harder before it feels easier. After all, you won't be responding to your baby's every cry by "simply" placing him on the breast (or bottle), but you will be taking the first steps toward raising a confident, respectable child who will respond positively to order and routine. I believe this is a gift that keeps on giving!

Here's what I want to make clear as well: There is no ONE right way to parent your baby. This book is a compilation of ideas and suggestions based on what worked for me, but I absolutely do not expect or want you to take these words as Biblical truths that must be followed to a tee. After all, your baby is not a robot, and neither are you! You are both unique individuals with your own personalities and you should make decisions based on what works for you. My goal is for you to have confidence in the decisions you choose and the ability to STICK WITH THEM. No more looking around and comparing yourself to all the other parents. No more second-guessing and mom guilt. It's time to equip ourselves with knowledge so we can have confidence in the choices that we make for our families.

Before we start to judge the choices of fellow parents, don't forget that we all share something very important in common: we all love our children and want what's best for them. Our methods for obtaining that may look different, but our hearts ultimately long for the same thing. If you don't want to implement some of the methods I advise, that is absolutely your choice. My hope is simply to give you tools that will empower you and your partner to make decisions that are unique to your child and his needs... decisions that are kind and loving but keep YOU in charge.

How to Read This Book

In Chapter 2, I will discuss many of the "Hot Topics" that new parents encounter in their baby's first year. If you are particularly prone to anxiety, you may wish to skip this section initially and refer back to it when related questions come up. If you like to know all the facts up front, this chapter will provide you with knowledge that will help you make informed decisions regarding the care of your baby.

Starting in Chapter 3, you will be led through a week-by-week, chronological guide to your baby's first year. Keep in mind that every baby is different, and these methods are never meant to increase stress with the expectation that it must be followed perfectly. It is organized this way so that you can approach each week with *one* main focus in mind rather than feel stuck and overwhelmed by trying to implement copious amounts of advice into any given day. Each chapter also includes "Other Topics on the Radar," which will address subjects and issues that may come up around that time frame.

It is also worth noting that the timeline of this information is based on healthy, full-term babies. If your baby was born prematurely, start Week One around his due date. If you are picking up this book after the birth of your baby, start at the beginning and read up until your baby's age, implementing the concepts along the way. If you would rather not follow along chronologically, use the "Contents" page to seek out topics that are relevant to you and your baby's needs. However, it is important to understand that these concepts are meant to build upon each other and I do not expect immediate success for someone who jumps months ahead without understanding the overall perspective.

If anything in this book rubs you the wrong way, listen to that! Skip to the next chapter, move on, answer to your own convictions and make a system that works for YOU. Start observing the families around you. Ask questions of the parents you admire and develop a plan that fits your personality and lifestyle.

Dearest parents-to-be, I am so proud of you. Weird, I know, because I don't know you, but I thought about you as I spent some sleepless nights (ironic?) writing these pages and I envisioned these words encouraging you and giving you hope. You are doing the hard work of equipping yourself with knowledge, and I completely believe this will enable you to thrive in parenthood and raise wonderful, well-rested children. I believe you have what it takes to become the next "Baby Sleep Boss." Let's get started!

- 1 -

GOALS OF THE BSB METHOD

For healthy, full-term babies who follow The BSB Method from birth, these are the realistic goals that you can expect to experience in your own home:

1. Your baby can sleep through the night (10-12 hours uninterrupted) by four months of age.

2. Your baby can establish a consistent nap routine during the day.

3. Your baby can learn to self-soothe and fall asleep independently, ideally without rocking or nursing.

4. Your baby can take a bottle so that both parents can work or enjoy free time away.

5. Your baby can be flexible enough to fall asleep at other people's houses, in pack-n-plays, and in other settings outside of his normal home environment.

6. You and your partner can approach parenting as a team and can both play a vital role in raising and sleep training your baby.

7. You can rest… you can thrive… you can become the very next "Baby Sleep Boss."

- 2 -

HOT TOPICS FOR NEW PARENTS

Before we jump into the weekly focus points you will implement once your new baby arrives, it's important to address some of the common topics you will encounter during these first few months of parenting. Many of these topics are controversial and there are arguments for and against each one, so clearly there is no right or wrong answer here. When making decisions regarding these topics, please remember that YOU are the boss. I will provide researched information for each one, as well as what worked for me. Do your homework, consult with your partner and pediatrician, and make a plan that aligns with your convictions. Then stick with it! These topics are not black and white, but they are YOUR decision.

SLEEP PROPS
Sleep props are any object or activity that aids your baby into falling asleep, such as rocking him to sleep,

nursing him to sleep, driving him around in the car, co-sleeping, etc. My encouragement is to avoid them completely or remove them within the first four months. My argument against sleep props is that when you develop a habit that allows your baby to depend on something to fall asleep, he will naturally continue to depend on that something in order to fall asleep. Makes sense, right? If that something is you nursing him to sleep every night and for every nap, guess where you will be every night and for every nap for the next year (or two) of your life? Guess where else you will be *in the middle of the night* when your baby wakes up? That's right - nursing your baby back to sleep! This may seem harmless in the beginning, but it is exhausting over the long haul, and it is completely avoidable if the habit is never initiated in the first place. What you allow is what you encourage.

I am also a huge advocate of my babies being able to sleep *anywhere* and to go down to sleep for *anyone*. For this reason, I minimized sleep props and had my babies taking naps all over the house (in a pack-n-play, crib or bassinet) within the first few weeks of life. This meant that if I ever had a girls' night out or a date night with my husband, a babysitter, grandparent, or literally any responsible adult could put our baby down to sleep *without us.* What freedom! In addition, we got our babies accustomed to sleeping at our friends' houses from an early age and this has literally saved us thousands of dollars over the years. To this day, all three of my children (ages one, three and five) will agreeably go to sleep at another house so my husband and I can enjoy time with our friends without having to hire a babysitter (or getting stuck at home every night!). When the time comes to go, we wake the kids up, quietly transfer them to their car seats, then transfer them straight to their beds once at home. People are surprised at our ability to do this, but it is possible if implemented early and consistently. Remember, you are the parent and you make the rules. Do this repeatedly with love and confidence and your children will learn to follow your lead.

When deciding on certain sleep props and whether or not you wish to use them, a good question to ask yourself is this: *Is the habit I am creating* sustainable *for me and my baby?* There are plenty of mothers who choose to co-sleep, nurse their babies to sleep, etc., and none of this is *wrong*; these are simply different strategies for raising children and not ones that I personally find freeing and life-giving. On the other hand, I welcome pacifiers and sound machines in my home and find that both are extremely beneficial in helping babies achieve deeper, longer sleep. By definition, both are considered sleep props, but both felt sustainable to my family and our needs.

CO-SLEEPING

Co-sleeping (often referred to as "bed-sharing") is the practice of parents and young children sleeping in the same bed. I won't spend a lot of time addressing this topic because I will say up-front that this was never entertained as an option in our home. Aside from the occasional morning snuggle time, our marriage bed is kept sacred and protected, and my husband and I don't feel badly about prioritizing our relationship and our own sleep needs in this way.

Some parents choose to co-sleep, whether out of choice for bonding, or out of desperation when their baby's night wakings become excessive. A baby who co-sleeps with his parents can still learn to be an adaptable sleeper who is able to self-soothe, but typically only when parents decide to move him to a crib in his own room.

Here are some important things to think about when deciding if co-sleeping is right for your family:

- What those in favor of co-sleeping say:
  - ○ Makes for more convenient nighttime nursing sessions.
  - ○ Helps your baby fall asleep faster after nighttime nursing sessions.
  - ○ Increases emotional bonds by promoting physical closeness.

- What those against co-sleeping say:
  - ○ Bed-sharing is a risk factor for Sudden Infant Death Syndrome (SIDS).[1]
  - ○ Research has shown that co-sleeping in infancy is associated with the later development of sleep problems.[2]
  - ○ Bed sharing in the first 6 months is associated with chronic night wakings for a baby.[3]
  - ○ Makes it difficult to teach your baby self-soothing techniques.
  - ○ Can be taxing on parents and interrupt their own sleep needs.

PACIFIERS

Some strict sleep training methods are completely against pacifier use as they are technically considered a "sleep prop," but, as mentioned previously, I support them. I found that with two of my three babies, a pacifier provided the oral stimulation that is normal and expected at this stage of life. Freud calls this the "Oral Phase" for a reason, and – when used correctly – I did not find that a pacifier interfered with my baby's ability to breastfeed or to fall asleep independently. Here are some pacifier pros and cons to help with your decision-making:

- Pacifier Pros:
    - Research has linked their use to a decreased risk of SIDS.[4]
    - Helps satiate a baby's need for non-nutritive sucking.
    - Helps a baby feel soothed and calmed in times of distress.
    - They're really stinkin' cute! Have you seen the little WubbaNub® animals?!

- Pacifier Cons:
    - A baby who relies on a pacifier to fall asleep will rely on YOU to provide his pacifier if he wakes up in the middle of the night. This gets easier when your baby is old enough to find his pacifier and put it back in his mouth himself, but it is pretty frustrating in the first few months.
    - Can be a challenging habit to break in toddler years.

- If you are too quick to offer a pacifier to your baby when he is crying, you might overlook the true reason for his cry (i.e. hunger, sickness, dirty diaper, etc.).
- Can cause issues of misaligned teeth and recurrent ear infections but typically only when used past 2 years of age.

SWADDLING

I found swaddling to be very helpful for my babies and their sleep habits, so my advice will be based in favor of swaddling (for the first 3 months). However, this is another decision that can go either way, so here is some information from both sides:

- What those in favor of swaddling say:
  - Creates a womb-like sensation and prevents a baby's jerking movements (startle reflex) from waking him up.
  - Helps babies feel calmer and sleep longer.
  - May help prevent SIDS because it encourages parents to put their baby to sleep on his back.

- What those against swaddling say:
  - It is unnecessary, and babies need to be able to move and put their hand in their mouth.

- ○ Can cause issues of overheating and/or altered circulation.
- ○ Creates a habit that may be difficult to break.
- ○ Can contribute to issues with hip dysplasia.

If you do decide to swaddle your baby, do so for naps and nighttime sleep, and unswaddle for feedings. I recommend using a large, square swaddle blanket that can achieve a tight, effective swaddle. There are great swaddling demonstrations online, so I suggest watching one so you can learn an effective method. The most important aspects are to keep your baby's arms straight down against his body, tuck and tighten with each maneuver, and give it some time. Some babies protest this initially but will eventually learn to associate this with sleep as it mimics the tight womb they are used to. In my experiences, this can make a huge difference in ushering your baby towards deep sleep that is unaffected by his startle reflex.

CRYING IT OUT

I will be the first to say that I have hated this term since the first time I heard it. It sounds awful and torturous, doesn't it? For me, there is a perspective shift that must take place. Think about it like this: *What is my ultimate goal here? Is my baby's* safety *in question or simply his* discomfort? *What are my own limitations and boundaries on how much crying I can handle?* With The BSB Method, there *will* be some crying involved, and I believe this is an inconvenient but necessary factor in sleep training.

I like to think about sleep the same way I think about diet and exercise. All three are necessary components of a healthy lifestyle, yet each require some discipline and training. You can't successfully run a marathon without training the same way you can't expect a baby to sleep through the night without some training. *Does training feel wonderful and breezy at all times?* Of course not! *Is my job to protect my baby from any discomfort in his life or is it to prepare him on how to handle the discomforts that life will inevitably bring?* This requires some hard work and commitment but all with the overall mentality of working toward your final goal of teaching your baby how to sleep.

Teaching a baby to sleep through the night will inevitably involve some tears, but the idea with The BSB Method is that, by implementing the sleep training strategies in a gradual manner and learning how to put your baby down to sleep before he is overtired, your baby will slowly adapt over time and will not require any "cold turkey" all-night cry fests.

23

Even so, listening to your baby cry can literally feel like stabbing daggers into your heart, so it's important to remember some of these truths about crying:

- Crying does not always mean that something is wrong with your baby. Crying is simply a baby's form of communication and it is his way of expressing pushback and resistance to something new. In some situations, his safety is in question and his crying most certainly needs to be addressed. In other situations, his comfort is in question, and his crying may or may not need to be addressed. It is your job as the parent to decide whether it is his *safety* or his *comfort* that is in question, and then respond accordingly (which may actually mean not responding at all!). If ever in doubt, ask yourself: *Is my baby unsafe or is he simply uncomfortable?*

- It is okay for your baby to cry. In a study of newborn babies at The Mayo Clinic, researchers found that the babies cried an average of 2-3 hours per day and much of this crying could not be attributed to any obvious cause.[5] Translation: all babies cry and that is normal! Subsequent studies have shown that "crying it out" does not have poor effects on a baby's stress (cortisol) levels or on their ability to bond with their parents.[6,7] All three of my boys required some periods of crying to learn how to sleep independently, yet they are all secure, loved, confident individuals without question.

- Every minute your baby cries will feel like an hour. That's not science... that's just mom truth. It is really, really hard to listen to your baby cry for extended periods of time. This is why I feel strongly in the teamwork with your partner here. Can you both be dedicated to the plan you have set in place? Is one of you more tolerant of crying than the other? Can you take a break and go for a walk while your baby cries and your partner stands guard?

- Research shows that babies with sleeping difficulties do not simply grow out of them, but rather these issues continue for roughly three to five years (WHAT?!).[8] While it is extremely difficult to listen to your infant cry, it would only be harder to hear your toddler screaming "Mooooommyyyyy!" at the top of his lungs throughout the night. You will be doing yourself a tremendous favor by implementing sleep strategies earlier in your child's life rather than later. It is much easier to *prevent* sleep issues than it is to *fix* them. Short-term pain, long-term gain!

Okay, I'm getting ahead of myself. We will revisit the topic of crying in Week Eight (Chapter 11) as you implement more concepts of sleep training for your baby.

SIDS PREVENTION

This is – without a doubt – my least favorite subject of all time to discuss. However, knowing the risks associated with Sudden Infant Death Syndrome (SIDS) is a necessity for all new parents. SIDS, by definition, is when a baby 12 months or younger dies during sleep with no warning signs or clear reason. Knowing the risk factors can help to ease your anxiety and provide safety measures toward prevention.

The American Academy of Pediatrics' (AAP) recommendations for preventing SIDS are:

- Always place your baby to sleep on his back – including naps and at night. If your baby rolls onto his stomach by himself, he may be left in that position.[9]

- Use a firm sleep surface with a tightly-fitting sheet.
- Keep soft objects and loose bedding out of the baby's sleep area. This means no blankies, lovies, frilly crib bumpers, etc. These can increase the risk of suffocation.
- Keep your baby's room temperature cool at 65-72 degrees Fahrenheit and do not overdress your baby (no more than one layer more than you are wearing).
- Share a room with your baby but never the same bed. (More about my take on this can be found in Chapter 8).
- Use a ceiling fan or floor fan to increase air circulation. This alone has been shown to decrease the risk of SIDS by 72 percent![10]
- Additional recommendations for SIDS reduction include the avoidance of exposure to smoke, alcohol, and illicit drugs; breastfeeding; routine immunization; and use of a pacifier.

Now that we have discussed some of the various facts and opinions that you will encounter over the next year, it's time to get started on your own game plan. Above all else, I hope you are enjoying some adorable newborn snuggles, soaking in every darling baby sigh, and finding that "sweet baby scent" amidst all the dirty diapers. Here we go!

- 3 -

WEEK ONE

PRIMARY FOCUS:

Help your baby get FULL FEEDINGS.

For the first two weeks of your baby's life, your number one job is to keep your baby awake at the breast (or bottle). This means that while your baby is feeding and constantly dozing off to La-La Land, your goal is to keep him awake so that he can get a full tummy with each feeding. This will be harder than you think and you won't always be successful, but keep in mind that this is an ideal to strive for and will simply take some practice.

Ideas for keeping your baby awake include: undressing him, massaging his legs, tickling his feet, changing his diaper, talking to him, etc.

Why is this important? When breastfeeding, there are

29

two types of milk expressed. Foremilk is the milk expressed at the beginning of a feeding. Think of this like skim milk. Hindmilk is the milk expressed at the end of a feeding and it is full of all the fat and good stuff. Think of this like whole milk. If a baby is fed every time he makes a sound, he is constantly getting that skim milk, falling asleep, then waking up hungry since he wasn't properly satiated in the first place. If you continue to allow this, he will develop a habit of snacking and he will need to feed more frequently, but he won't be taking in the fatty milk he really needs. If you can keep your baby from falling asleep during a feeding, he will make his way to the whole milk, fill up his tummy, develop adorable, squishy rolls, and make it much longer until the next feeding. Woohoo! This goes for formula-fed babies as well. Either way, a full tummy with each feeding is the goal.

- For the first few weeks of your baby's life, you will feed your baby an average of eight to ten feedings a day and each feeding will last around 30-45 minutes (roughly 15-20 minutes on each side with burping in between). If your baby nurses less frequently, only nurses for 10 minutes or less, or you hear a clicking sound during nursing, you may want to consider utilizing a local lactation consultant to make sure your baby is latching on and feeding properly.

- Feedings will occur every 1 ½ to 2 hours from the *start* of one feeding to the *start* of the next. Yes, this is as exhausting as it sounds, but hang in there, sister! It is short-lived! Your baby should transition naturally into a 2 ½- to 3-hour routine within two weeks.

Note: For night feedings, wait a few minutes to respond to make sure it's a true hunger cry (babies are really noisy sleepers!). Set a timer if this helps you, with a good rule of thumb being *at least* 1 minute per week of age (i.e. At 2 weeks of age, wait 2 minutes before responding to your baby's cry; at 3 weeks of age, wait 3 minutes, and so on). That being said, please don't let this create anxiety in you. I am not actually suggesting that you pull out a timer every time your baby cries and say, "Okay, my baby is 4 weeks old… set the timer for 4 minutes!" The whole idea is to practice delaying your response as a way of teaching your baby self-soothing techniques. It's also a way for you to gain confidence in the reality that some crying will not do your baby any harm. Just ask second and third babies who don't have the luxury of instant gratification. They are notoriously more "chill" and independent, and I believe this is because they have had to learn these skills earlier due to their parents' attention being stretched elsewhere.

OTHER TOPICS ON THE RADAR

SKIN-TO-SKIN CONTACT

Skin-to-skin contact is the practice of laying a baby on his mother or father's bare chest. There is growing evidence that skin-to-skin contact after birth has numerous benefits for parents and their baby, aiding in bonding, milk production, calming the baby, regulating the baby's heart rate, and even stimulating digestion.[1] Simply strip your baby down to his diaper and lay him directly on your chest. Enjoy these sweet moments and try to cherish every baby noise and sigh because this season is precious but gone in a blink. These chest naps are heaven!

MILK COMING IN

For the first few days of your baby's life, he will take in a secretion from the mammary glands called colostrum, which is thick, yellow, super-nutritious and rich in antibodies. The official breastmilk usually comes in between days 3-5, so get ready to go from double-A to a double-D, ladies! For real, this can be quite impressive and is often associated with discomfort, lethargy, night sweats, hot flashes, and lots of other fun, hormoney symptoms. Oh, the joys! During that period, some weight loss in the baby (up to 10 percent of birth weight) is normal and expected to be regained within 10 days.[2]

After your milk comes in, you may feel a pressure and tingling sensation in your nipples within the first few minutes of nursing. This is called the "let-down reflex" and it signifies that your hormones are doing their job of filling your breasts with plenty of milk for your baby. Let-down usually happens simultaneously in both breasts, so you'll want to use a nursing pad or silicone breast pump to catch the leakage from the breast you aren't using.

Note: If your let-down is particularly forceful and your baby seems to be choking, make sure the entire areola (brown circle around your nipple) is in his mouth and he has a good latch (see more in Breastfeeding Basics). If this continues, pull him off, hand-express some milk into a towel, and try nursing again.

CLUSTER FEEDING

Sometime in the first week of your baby's life you will experience a night (or two) that is marked with your baby's constant desire to feed. This can literally look like feedings every hour for roughly 45 minutes at a time and you will want to cry and crawl in a hole and never come out. With my first baby I tracked this insanity with a nursing app and found that my baby nursed for something like 13 hours in a 24-hour period. WHAT IN THE WORLD?! This is physically and emotionally taxing and it's no wonder that my nipples turned to hamburger meat in no time. Had I known that this thing had a name and wasn't just some cruel trick sent by Satan himself, I would've handled it with a little more grit. Important things to remember during this grueling period are:

- This is short-lived and necessary to establish your milk production.

- This can also rear its ugly head during your baby's growth spurts, which typically occur around 2-3 weeks, 5-7 weeks, 3 months, 6 months, 9 months, and 12 months. YAY!

- It is important to protect your nipples during this time in any way you can.

BOSS tip: Think of your breastmilk as a healing salve and express a little onto your nipples after each feeding. Seriously, that stuff is liquid GOLD. Additionally, invest in a good nipple cream (like lanolin) and consider wearing nipple shields under your bra to prevent rubbing... whatever you can find that is helpful to keep those things intact!

BREASTFEEDING BASICS

Breastfeeding is a wonderful, beautiful way to aid in health and bonding with your baby, but it can also be very HARD. Everyone made me feel like this was going to be a breezy thing that came naturally to me so when I faced issues of any kind I felt shameful and anxious. If breastfeeding doesn't come easily to you and your baby, don't panic! There is nothing wrong with you. This is a process that you and your baby will learn together, and it may just take some practice.

Try to keep in mind that the demands of breastfeeding will be most taxing in the first few months of your baby's life. If you are able to persevere through this period, you will be relieved to discover that breastfeeding gets a whole lot easier when your baby can nurse more efficiently, stretch out his feedings, and sleep through the night. You got this, sister!

First of all, how do I actually DO it? Start by placing your baby on your lap and tilting his body to face you. If you are starting on the right side, hold your breast with your right hand, support your baby's head with your left hand, and adjust your position until his mouth can make contact with your nipple. This is called the "cradle hold" and can be made easier by using a nursing pillow. If you have particularly large breasts or had to have a C-section, you may prefer the "football hold," where your baby is cradled along your side facing you, with his legs tucked under your arm on the same side you are nursing from (literally like holding a football). There are a number of different positions you can use while breastfeeding and one is not better than the other, so give it a whirl and find the one that feels most natural to you. Other favorites are the side-lying position and the laid-back position.

When your baby's mouth makes contact with your nipple and it forms a good suction, this is called the "latch." In order to get a good latch, aim your nipple toward the baby's upper lip, rub it along his lip, and keep your fingers clear from the area. Once he makes contact, you should feel a little pressure and discomfort, and your baby should start sucking. If you have pain, hear a clicking sound, or it appears that your baby is not swallowing, slide your little finger between your breast and the corner of your baby's mouth to break the suction, then try again until he gets it. If you continue to have issues, seek out help from a lactation consultant. Getting a good latch is crucial to establish breastfeeding and can wreak havoc on your nipples if done improperly. Once you've got it going, take a sigh of relief. You're really doing it! You're breastfeeding a baby! Isn't it surreal and amazing?!

Now it's time to keep that baby awake and start to monitor his feedings. I found it helpful to keep track of feedings using a nursing app (such as BabyConnect) and this will help you remember which side you started on with the previous feeding. As recommended to me by a lactation consultant, I approached breastfeeding like this: I would feed my baby on the right breast for 10-15 minutes (or until the breast feels soft and empty), burp him, feed him on the left breast for 10-15 minutes (or until the baby seems content), burp him again, change his diaper, then prepare him for his nap. After he woke up from his nap I would start feeding on the side I finished on last (in this example, the left side), which seems contradictory but helps with stimulating milk production equally on both sides. It is normal for one breast to produce more than the other, but this will help your baby develop a habit of fully emptying on both sides.

Here are some helpful breastfeeding tid-bits to lighten your load:

- In the first few weeks post-partum, your uterus will continue to contract during nursing as your body releases oxytocin, a hormone associated with bonding activities like birth, breastfeeding, and sex. Remember all those crampy periods you missed over the past 9 months? Well, they'll show up like one huge period over the next few weeks as you cramp and bleed. What fun! Not to worry though; this is a normal finding and a good indicator that your uterus is shrinking back to its old self and preventing further bleeding.

- Increase your caloric intake by about 300-500 calories a day to make enough milk for your baby, particularly in the first few months of breastfeeding. Try to make the calories count by incorporating plenty of fresh fruits, vegetables, and whole grains into your diet. Continue taking your daily prenatal vitamin, as this will help to fill in any nutritional gaps on those days when all you want is ice cream (and believe me, I've been there!).

- If you are having trouble producing enough milk, consider adding these lactogenic foods into your diet to help increase your milk supply: almonds, leafy greens, fennel seeds, oats, apricots, dates, legumes, and brewer's yeast. Most natural grocery stores also have supplements made specifically for milk production. And don't forget to drink lots and lots of water!

Note: If you develop any localized redness, lumps, or pain on either of your breasts, you could be developing a plugged milk duct. Take a hot shower, massage the area, self-express milk from that side, and continue nursing your baby or pumping during this time (even though this will be painful). Take Ibuprofen to minimize the pain and swelling. Notify your doctor right away if you develop a fever or generalized achiness, as this may indicate that an infection called mastitis has developed, and this requires treatment with antibiotics.

- If you like to indulge in an alcoholic beverage from time to time, try to drink it while nursing or soon thereafter, as studies have shown that it takes roughly 3 hours for alcohol to be cleared from your breastmilk.[3]

- Foods that notoriously cause gas in babies are beans, broccoli, brussels sprouts, cabbage, cauliflower, prunes, citrus fruits, spicy foods, caffeine, and excessive amounts of dairy.

- If your baby is particularly gassy/fussy, consider your diet and any medications you take. If you or your baby have had to be on an antibiotic for any reason, this could be affecting your baby's GI system and you may want to consider starting an oral probiotic for him and/or yourself.

- If your baby seems mostly content *except when nursing*, it might be time to seek out some help. This could be an issue of your milk supply or your baby's ability to latch. Alternately, some babies develop reflux issues that can be treated with over-the-counter medications which can make a world of a difference. Pediatricians and lactation consultants are excellent resources that you should utilize if your baby is facing any feeding difficulties.

Oh breastfeeding... doesn't this all sound so fun and natural? Well, I'm so proud of you for giving this a shot and I hope that you and your baby will find a rhythm together in no time.

Note to the non-breastfeeders: If you aren't able to breastfeed, please don't beat yourself up about it! Every mom-baby combo will have their fair share of issues and if breastfeeding just isn't your thing, you should never be made to feel bad about that. If you line up a group of kindergarten students, I am certain that you wouldn't be able to distinguish which children were breastfed and which ones weren't. Your baby will be JUST FINE. I will address breastfeeding moms throughout the text, but it is never meant to make any non-breastfeeding moms feel guilty or less-than.

- 4 -

WEEK TWO

PRIMARY FOCUS:

Set up a routine with three activities in this order: EAT, PLAY, SLEEP.

Your days will be made up of a repetitive cycle consisting of these three steps:

1. You will feed your baby (EAT)
2. You will bond with your baby and keep him awake (PLAY)
3. You will swaddle your baby and put him down to rest (SLEEP)

When your baby wakes up, you will repeat the process. This routine provides a consistent daily rhythm, helps to maintain your milk supply, and encourages longer stretches of sleep for your baby at night.

> **Note:** The exception to this routine is the nighttime feedings in which you would NOT want to encourage any "Play" time. Skip this step and lay your baby back down after he has been fed, burped, changed and re-swaddled.

1. **EAT**: Feeding time will be roughly 20-30 minutes and will occur every 2 to 2 ½ hours from the *start* of one feeding to the *start* of the next. For breastfeeding moms, this means that you will be feeding 10-15 minutes on one side, burping him, then feeding 10-15 minutes on the other side.

    *   **Signs of hunger:** crying, smacking his lips, sucking on his fists, and rooting.

    *   For the first month of age, your baby should average 8-10 feedings in a 24-hour period.[1] He should take in a total of 20-24 ounces of breastmilk or formula per day, which averages roughly 2-3 ounces per feeding. From 2-3 months of age, this becomes roughly 24-32 ounces over 6-8 feedings per day, each averaging 4-6 ounces. Some babies will take a little more; some will take a little less. Monitor your baby's wet and

dirty diapers and notify your pediatrician if you have any concerns.

- If your baby sleeps longer than 2 ½ hours during the day, wake him up for his next feeding to keep him on a routine. Yes, I know, "You never wake a sleeping baby," but with The BSB Method, I beg to differ. Babies are naturally searching for a longer chunk of sleep and if you let this happen during the day, this is when it will continue to happen. In addition, waking a baby to feed him is important for establishing your milk production and ensuring that your baby receives enough nutrition during the day. It is your job to teach him how to solidify a daily feeding routine so that he relies on the day time for eating and the night time for sleeping. After the late evening feeding (around 10pm), let your baby sleep as long as he allows. (Some resources will encourage you to wake him after 5 hours to keep your lactation steady, but I never did this. You would certainly want to consider this if you are having issues with milk supply and/or if your baby is having issues with gaining weight).

Note: I am obviously a big fan of the Eat-Play-Sleep routine and feel strongly that this naturally creates a good sleep rhythm for babies. However, there will most certainly be times when you can and should deviate from this order. If your baby is sick or going through a growth spurt, his feeding demands will increase and he may require an extra feeding before his nap (or in the middle of it) to soothe him into sleep. This is not wrong! Likewise, if you are traveling and putting your baby down to sleep at a different time or in a new setting, his feeding schedule may look a little different. Use your judgement and act in confidence. When the illness subsides or you return from vacation, reimplement his normal sleep habits and expect 1-3 days to get your baby back on track.

2. **PLAY**: Work towards keeping your baby awake for 45 minutes in the beginning (including feeding time), then slowly stretch out this time as your baby is able.

- For the first 3 months, feeding + play/awake time should last roughly 1 hour or less, as your baby can get overtired and overstimulated, then NOT be able to sleep. From 3-5 months, play/awake time can last 1-2 hours, then continue to stretch out in the following months. Watch your baby for signs of drowsiness while being mindful of the time and you will learn how to get your baby down to sleep before he becomes overtired.

- **Ideas for Play:** reading books, singing songs, laying your baby in a floor gym or a bouncer, tummy time, looking out the window, bath time, anything that promotes bonding with your baby!

- I am adamantly against any television or screen time for babies at this age. The AAP recommends NO screen time until 18 months of age, as this can cause overstimulation and alter brain development in babies.[2]

> **Note:** I was pretty good about this for my first baby but not as strict with the second. My older son had fallen madly in love with Daniel Tiger by then... how was I supposed to take that away?! All I'm saying is, be wise about this. Don't set your newborn baby in a bouncer facing the tv screen as a form of entertainment or distraction for him.

3. **SLEEP**: Naptime should be the last half of the cycle; then your baby will wake up ready to eat and repeat the process! In the beginning, naps can be roughly 1 to 1 ½ hours, then stretch to 1 ½ to 2 hours by 3 months of age.

- **Signs of drowsiness:** yawning, closing his fists, fluttering eyelids, difficulty focusing, grimacing, pulling at his ears, and jerking his arms and legs. If you see these signs in your baby and/or he has been awake between 1-2 hours, it is time to prepare him for sleep and stay ahead of the meltdown.

- **Signs of being overtired (melting down):** irritability, arching backwards, fussiness, rubbing his eyes, and hysterical crying. These are signals that you have missed the ideal time to put your baby down to sleep, and you may want to intervene 15-30 minutes earlier with the next cycle. No need to fret though! Remember that this is a process that the whole family is learning together and it was never meant to look perfect.

- Within the first few weeks of your baby's life, put him down for some of his naps in a crib, bassinet, or pack-n-play. It will be tempting to hold your baby or put him in a swing, bouncer, or car seat for all of his naps and this is certainly okay from time to time. However, early introduction to the crib will help your baby become an adaptable sleeper and will make him less reluctant to accept this as his sleep environment in the coming months. He probably won't love this at first, but keep in mind that this is one of the first steps to teaching him how to sleep independently. This will work best if you stay ahead of the meltdown and provide an optimal sleep setting.

- **Encouraged sleep components:** dark room, loud white noise, tightly swaddled, mesh crib bumpers, room temperature of 65-72 degrees, pacifier.

- **Discouraged sleep components:** flashy/musical mobile, blankets, stuffed animals, night lights, fluffy crib bumpers.

- For the first month, your baby is expected to sleep roughly sixteen to eighteen hours per day. They are basically like little sloths! He will take six to eight naps during a 24-hour period according to this Eat-Play-Sleep routine, and this will lessen over time as the intervals stretch out from one feeding to the next. This may seem excessive but sleep begets sleep! A baby who naps well during the day will be more prone to sleep better through the night.[3]

- It is worth mentioning that some babies will easily fall into a nap routine and some will not. Because babies are unique individuals and not robots, don't panic if your baby's nap schedule does not follow along perfectly. Some babies love naps... some babies are short nappers. The most important indicator of a rested baby is one who appears happy and content.

- If your baby is not napping well, consider cutting back on his play/awake time by 15-minute increments. It could be that he is staying awake too long, becoming fatigued and overstimulated, then fighting off sleep through crying.[4]

- Keep in mind that a baby's sleep cycle is around 30-45 minutes.[5] In this early period, your baby may wake and cry out during this time, but this doesn't necessarily mean he is ready to end his nap. Instead, leave him alone for a few minutes to see if he will settle himself back to sleep. Remember that naps at this stage can last roughly 1 ½ to 2 hours, so try to give your baby the chance to complete each Eat-Play-Sleep cycle by not rushing to him and feeding him at his every whimper.

I love this rhythm for so many reasons. First and foremost, it gives you a sense of control and predictability over your baby and the outline of your day. I loved that within the first few weeks of my baby's life, I could feed him, then leave him with my husband and go to the grocery store or run an errand to Target, knowing in confidence that I had approximately 1 ½ to 2 hours before I was needed again for a feeding. Because my husband was a good teammate with the Eat-Play-Sleep routine, he knew to keep the baby awake after the feeding, then put him down for a nap when he started to show signs of drowsiness. This rhythm provided freedom for me and empowerment for my husband. Our baby was safe and loved by both parents and our partnership thrived. Plus, I found some great new shirts at Target - WIN!

Note: While I never wanted to make myself a slave to my baby's schedule, I found that having a consistent routine provided me with incredible confidence in social settings. If my baby started crying but had just been fed 30 minutes earlier, I could kindly ignore the comments prompting me to feed him: "Oh he's crying... must be hungry!" Instead, I would burp him, check his diaper, then prepare him for sleep, either in his car seat or in a pack-n-play if available.

TROUBLESHOOTING

Once your baby establishes a rhythm on this Eat-Play-Sleep routine, you will notice somewhat of a consistent trend around what times he feeds every day. While it is important to be mindful of the natural schedule he is creating, you will also find that the timing of one of his activities will interfere with your own schedule from time to time. This is where consistency will pay off. Because his norm is routine, he will be able to flex where needed.

For example, if you have an appointment at 10:30am but you sense that he will be due for a feeding around this time, you have a few options: 1) You can pump right before you need to leave and have a bottle ready for your partner or a sitter, who can then feed your baby when he wakes up, 2) You can wake him up early from his nap and feed him so you can get to your appointment on time, or 3) You can put him down for that nap in his car seat, then leave for your appointment 20-30 minutes early and feed your baby when you arrive. Any of these may interfere a bit with his "normal" schedule, but as long as you continue with his Eat-Play-Sleep routine then it will all even out over the course of the day.

OTHER TOPICS
ON THE RADAR

DIAPERING

In the first three months of your baby's life, you will change his diaper an average of 8 to 10 times per day. This process may feel awkward and frustrating in the beginning, but you will quickly discover that you have plenty of opportunities to practice this skill. For the first month alone, you can expect 5-8 wet diapers and 3-4 stools on a daily basis. WOW!

Here are some diaper-changing tips and tricks to make you a pro in no time:

- Change your baby's diaper on a flat, steady surface and never leave him unattended. Babies can roll off a changing table long before they show this skill elsewhere.

- Choose a diaper brand that fits your lifestyle and budget. Some choose disposable diapers for their convenience and ease of use; others opt for cloth diapers in hopes of saving some dollars and the environment. There is no right or wrong decision!

- Use unscented, alcohol-free wipes and always wipe from front to back. Clean carefully between the skin folds, making sure not to leave any remnants that could cause irritation.

BOSS tip (for boy moms): Keep a clean, dry washcloth handy during diaper changes and lay it on top of your baby's boy parts to prevent yourself from getting showered.

- Coat your baby's bum with Vaseline®, Aquaphor® or another protective ointment after every diaper change as a means of preventing diaper rash from developing. If diaper rash does develop, leave your baby's bum open to air for a few minutes after each diaper change and then coat it with coconut oil or a zinc oxide-based cream, such as Boudreaux's Butt Paste®.

- Pack plenty of diapers in the diaper bag and always have a spare set of clothes with you. If you're unfamiliar with the term "blow-out," you're sure to discover it in no time!

- If using disposable diapers, invest in a good scent-containing diaper pail, such as The Diaper Genie®.

- Encourage your partner to participate in diaper changes and don't nitpick about his ability or system. Even if your baby's diaper is put on backwards, this doesn't affect his safety or well-being. Be forgiving toward others in their methods and welcome any help that is available.

> **BOSS tip:** As a way of making diaper changes more enjoyable for your baby, hang a musical mobile over his changing table. This is a great distraction for him and also stimulates play time!

BATHING

Your baby's umbilical cord stump should fall off between 1 to 3 weeks of age. Can I get a *Hallelujah*? That thing is weird and gross. After the stump falls off, you can give your baby his first real bath. Camera's ready!

Your baby may not love bath time at first, but utilize this time to bond with him, massage his cute, little body, and come up with a fun bath time song to sing to him. Wet babies are super slippery, so it is always best to utilize the help of your partner until you get the hang of this.

A newborn's bath does not have to be long or involved, but there are some important things to keep in mind:

- This can take place in a baby bath tub or the kitchen sink. If bathing in a sink, pad the bottom with a towel to make it softer and more comfortable.

- Gather all necessary items before getting started, as you should never leave your baby unattended near water. You will need: baby soap, a washcloth, a baby brush, a plastic cup, and a hooded towel.

- Test the temperature of the water with the back of your wrist or your elbow. The water should feel warm but not hot. You only need a few inches of water to get the job done.

- Cradle his head and neck and scrub between his fingers and toes, behind his ears, in those luscious skin folds along his thighs, under his chin, and in his little private parts. If he has hair, use a little baby soap or shampoo to massage into his scalp. If he has cradle cap (those weird scales on the top of his head), use a baby brush to gently exfoliate it away. If the cradle cap continues, put baby oil on his head one hour before his next bath as this will help to soften the scales so they can be wiped away.

- Keep the room temperature warm and utilize a space heater afterwards to keep him happy during his post-bath rub down. Pat his skin dry, focusing on the skin folds and private parts, and use a mild baby lotion as needed. Put on a fresh diaper and set of clothes, then take a big whiff of your baby. This is the "sweet newborn scent" you've always heard about, and it is heavenly!

Bathe your baby 2-3 times a week, or whenever you notice the need. A good way to check for cleanliness is to smell under his chin on the front of his neck where spit-up loves to accumulate. Trust me... you'll know if it's time for a bath!

SPITTING UP & BURPING

Some babies spit up a lot... some babies hardly spit up at all. This causes anxiety for a lot of new parents, especially when it seems like their baby is spitting up an entire feeding (which they rarely do!). This is why it's important to understand that spitting up is common in healthy babies and is not a cause for concern as long as your baby is eating well and gaining weight.[6] A few things you can do to minimize spitting up are:

- Burp your baby well during and after his feedings.

    o   In bottle feeding, this means you will burp your baby when he is roughly three-fourths of the way through his bottle, and then again when he is finished. In breastfeeding, this means you will burp your baby after he has emptied your breast on one side, then again after he seems content after nursing on the other side.

> **BOSS tip:** Try patting your baby on his lower back rather than on the upper back in order to express trapped gas from his tummy.

- Keep your baby somewhat upright during his feedings. If you are breastfeeding, prop his head up against your breast on the side he is eating from and let the rest of his body lay at a downward angle against your body. Keep him upright for the next 30 minutes if possible, and avoid any bouncing or swinging activities.

- Try not to overfeed him. This goes for breast- and bottle-feeding. Follow his cues that show he is full and don't force down another ounce for the sake of finishing off the bottle.

- Reevaluate your own diet. See "Breastfeeding Basics" in Chapter 3 for foods that can cause gas. Even though true dairy allergies are uncommon in babies, I did find that minimizing my dairy intake significantly helped to reduce reflux for one of my babies.

- Know when it's vomiting versus spitting up. Vomiting occurs when the baby's entire meal is brought back up forcefully, shooting out inches rather than just dribbling down his face. If your baby experiences frequent vomiting, contact your pediatrician.

You know your baby best. If anything about his eating or spitting up is concerning to you, don't hesitate to notify your pediatrician. Rest assured that most babies stop spitting up by 12 months and this is simply just his rite of passage into toddlerhood!

WEEK THREE

PRIMARY FOCUS:

Start pumping and giving your baby a bottle.

I will tell you this straight-up without beating around the bush: this is not the most fun part of breastfeeding. Pumping gets a bad rap for a reason. It can be frustrating, time-consuming, and may make you feel like an actual cow, but I believe it is a necessary part of motherhood if you wish to experience some personal freedom while breastfeeding. If you ever want to be away from your baby for more than a few hours at a time (which I highly recommend), I advise that you start pumping and giving your baby a bottle around his 2nd or 3rd week of life.

What does this look like? For pumping, I picked a time that could be somewhat consistent from day to day so that my body's supply-and-demand system could adjust accordingly. For baby number one, this was around 10am. Your milk supply will be greater in the morning hours so picking a morning time is advisable, but let's be realistic here. With baby number two, I had a two-year-old running around at 10am, so sitting quietly and calmly with my breast pump for 20 minutes was not an option. That go around, I chose 2pm when my older son would be napping and I could fit in a sufficient pumping session.

Pick a time that works for you. Feed your newborn, get him settled in a comfortable and safe spot, then pump until you are empty. Store this milk in a refrigerator or freezer for later use as you are able, but also – VERY IMPORTANT – start offering your baby a bottle with breastmilk around this 2- to 3-week mark.

BOSS tip: Record your baby crying and play this out loud to yourself when you are first trying to pump. This can stimulate the release of oxytocin and encourage your milk to let down.

For the first bottle feeding, have your partner or a family member give the baby his bottle and relish in a few minutes of rest. (But don't forget that you still have to pump for that missed feeding - RATS! See, I told you, breastfeeding is no joke!). Use the bottle of your choosing and make sure you have the correct nipple size in place. The nipples are sorted by age range to produce the amount of flow needed for your baby at that stage, so this is important. Provide a quiet and calm environment, squirt a few drops of milk on his lips to pique his interest, then offer your baby the bottle. Some babies take a bottle without any issues whatsoever; others put up a fuss and require many attempts and nipple types before they will relent. Be patient, calm and persistent until he gets it. Burp your baby after he has taken 2-3 ounces, then offer the bottle again. Continue this process until he seems content, then finish with a good final burp. Well done, everyone!

> **Note:** When starting a baby on formula, he may seem gassy and fussy until his body gets the hang of it. A baby's digestive system takes time to adjust to new enzymes and sugars found in formula, so I suggest sticking with the same formula for 5-7 days before changing to another brand or type.

Okay, so your baby took a bottle - YAY! Here's the kicker: do not set the bottle aside and not attempt this again until the week before you go back to work. You might find – to a lot of moms' surprise – that your baby no longer takes the bottle and you are *stuck*. That being said, you will want to start offering your baby a bottle around 2-3 weeks of age and then continue to offer it once a day *every 1-3 days*. This does take a bit of extra work, but it will make your life easier in the long haul when you can enjoy full days at work or even a weekend away with your girl friends. Now we're talking!

BREASTMILK STORING & THAWING

Until you get the hang of this, it will feel like 90% of your thoughts from day-to-day are focused on MILK…how to make it and what to do with it. Here is some helpful information to make this process smoother:

- When storing and thawing breastmilk, here are the timing guidelines:
  - May be stored in a refrigerator for 72 hours after pumping.
  - May be stored in a freezer (5-15 degrees Fahrenheit) for up to 3 months.

o   May be stored in a deep freezer (0 degrees Fahrenheit and below) for up to 6 months.

o   May be stored in a refrigerator for 24 hours after thawing frozen milk. Never refreeze thawed milk.

- Store the milk in increments of 1, 2, 3, or 4 ounces. As your baby ages, the amount of milk he takes with each feeding will fluctuate, so I liked having an option when it came to feeding time. If my baby typically took 4 ounces, I would thaw a 4-ounce bag, knowing in confidence that I had a 1- or 2-ounce bag available if he still seemed hungry.

- Store the milk laying down flat so that it will freeze this way. When it comes time to thaw, this is much quicker than thawing a large ball of milk (in bags stored upright).

- When thawing breastmilk, you can thaw it overnight in a refrigerator, run it under warm water, or let it rest in a mug filled with warm water. Never microwave breastmilk or let it thaw at room temperature.

- After the milk is completely thawed and free of any ice chunks, transfer it to the bottle and prepare your baby for his feeding.

OTHER TOPICS ON THE RADAR

THE WITCHING HOUR

Unbeknownst to most new parents, almost all babies have a period of the day when they are particularly fussy and hard to console. This is known as "the witching hour" and usually occurs in the late afternoon or evening hours. For all three of my boys, this delightful period almost always showed up between 5pm to 9pm. After having somewhat of a "normal," smooth day, my baby would start crying out of the blue and would remain inconsolable for 30 minutes to an hour. Wouldn't you know that this was almost always the time when a friend would want to stop by after work to meet the little guy or bring us a meal?! "I promise he isn't usually this fussy!" I'd proclaim anxiously. What I learned in time is that the witching hour is a perfectly normal phenomenon. It does not mean that something is wrong with your baby or that he has colic. Some evenings will be worse than others. Try to remain calm, offer your baby a bath or a walk in the stroller, bounce with him on an exercise ball, or give him a massage. Utilize your partner to tag-team the situation and give each other breaks as you are able.

For most babies, the witching hour eases over time and vanishes completely around three months of age. If your baby's evening fussiness continues past three months, this is a good indicator that he may be short on sleep and you will want to focus your efforts on good daytime naps to keep him from getting overtired.

COLIC

Colic is a difficult diagnosis to pinpoint because nearly all new moms think at some point that their baby is colicky. Don't forget that crying is normal and less than 20% of babies actually have colic. According to Dr. Marc Weissbluth in *Healthy Sleep Habits, Happy Child*, an official diagnosis of colic is assumed when a healthy, well-fed baby meets these three criteria:

1. Your baby cries for a total of more than three hours per day.
2. This occurs more than three days in any one week.
3. This has been occurring for more than three weeks.

If you are currently checking yes to the first two questions and start seeing the third yes in the coming weeks, first of all, I am so sorry. Having a colicky baby can be taxing on parents and often leads to feelings of isolation and desperation. Utilize your partner and any extra, trustworthy hands you can find. You have done nothing wrong and this does not mean you don't love your baby or that you aren't capable of raising him well. The strategies for teaching self-soothing may need to take a backseat at this time and that is perfectly okay. Your baby is likely going to need to be "parent-soothed" during this period until the colic subsides, which usually takes place around 2 months and then completely resolves around 4 months. Hang in there!

SOOTHING TECHNIQUES

Whether your baby is colicky or not, it is imperative to understand that all babies cry and can't always be consoled. However, I found that Harvey Karp's "Happiest Baby" methods were really helpful in times of desperation. His "5 S's" for soothing a crying baby are:

1. **Swaddle:** Wrap your baby tightly in a large, square swaddling blanket with his arms straight against his sides and his hips loose and flexed. This recreates the security of a womb-like environment.

2. **Side or Stomach position:** Hold your baby on his side, on his stomach, or over your shoulder. This puts gentle pressure on his tummy and can relieve gastrointestinal upset.

3. **Shush:** Use your voice or white noise to mimic the loud humming noises your baby was used to in the womb.

4. **Swing:** Support your baby's head/neck, hold him tightly against your body and provide swift, tiny motions back and forth. I also found it effective to gently bounce with my baby on an exercise ball or to "swing" my baby in a gentle Figure-8 motion.

5. **Suck:** Offer your baby his finger or a pacifier for non-nutritive sucking.

Other helpful methods for soothing your little one include:

- **Infant Massage:** this is the practice of gently stroking and kneading your baby's body to encourage bonding and soothing. Wait at least 45 minutes after a feeding to give this a try.

- **Exercise Ball:** hold your baby tightly and gently bounce with him on an exercise ball until he is calm.

- **"The Plus Sign":** move your thumb gently and slowly across your baby's forehead and down his nose, making a plus sign. Repeat this movement until your baby is calm and relaxed.

There are unlimited strategies for soothing a crying baby, but with a little experimentation and practice, you will learn your baby and his preferences in no time!

WEEK FOUR

PRIMARY FOCUS:

Evaluate the routine you are creating.

Your baby should be transitioning into a 2 ½- to 3-hour routine at this point (from the *start* of one feeding to the *start* of the next).

What if he's not stretching out his routine? Ask yourself some questions:

- *Am I feeding him immediately when he starts crying, even though his cry could mean something else? Could he be too hot or too cold, have a dirty diaper, or simply need a change of scenery?*

- *Am I keeping my baby awake during his feedings so that he gets a full tummy each time?*

- *Are my partner and I working together as a team in the Eat-Play-Sleep routine?*

- *Do I need to consult extra help from a lactation consultant or a baby sleep consultant* (such as The Baby Sleep Boss, wink wink!)?

Sample Schedule (2 ½ - 3-hour routine)

For this sample schedule, keep in mind that your baby's feeding times will be quite fluid from day-to-day for the first two months of his life. Observe this schedule as a guide to follow for the rhythm of your day, but don't expect to be able to implement any set feeding times at this point.

Early AM (6:00am)	Wake up, feeding, diaper change, play/awake time, nap
Mid-AM (9:00am)	Feeding, diaper change, play/awake time, nap
Late AM (11:30am)	Feeding, diaper change, play/awake time, nap
Mid-Afternoon (2:30pm)	Feeding, diaper change, play/awake time, nap

Late Afternoon (5:00pm)	Feeding, diaper change, play/awake time, nap
Early PM (7:30pm)	Feeding, diaper change, play/awake time, nap
Late PM (10:00pm)	Feeding, diaper change, pj's, swaddle, down for the night
During the Night (1-3 times)	Feeding, diaper change, re-swaddle, then immediately back down for the night

TROUBLESHOOTING

Some parents report that they have a difficult time getting their baby down for a nap between the Early PM and Late PM feedings. In this case, I would suggest keeping your baby awake after his Early PM feeding, then feeding him again for his Late PM feeding within 2 to 2 ½ hours of his previous feeding, and then preparing him for bed as you see signs of drowsiness. This fills up his tummy to allow for a longer stretch of night sleep, and it keeps him from staying awake too long and becoming overstimulated.

Other parents report that their baby falls asleep after the Early PM feeding and is difficult to wake for the

Late PM feeding. Here you have a few options:

1. You can treat this as bedtime and put your baby down for the night at this earlier hour (around 7:30pm). Then you may wish to go to bed shortly thereafter so you can catch some sleep before his next feeding.

2. You can wake your baby around 10:00pm to offer another feeding (sometimes called a "dream feed"). Your baby may be really sleepy during this feeding, but try to keep him awake and get him a full tummy before putting him right back down to bed for the night. Then you can both go to bed.

3. You can feed your baby the Early PM feeding, pump shortly thereafter, and prepare a bottle for your partner to give whenever your baby wakes up next. Then you can go to bed at an earlier hour (around 8pm) and catch a longer stretch of sleep until your baby wakes up during the night for a feeding.

My husband and I did a combination of all three options depending on each baby and his unique needs. I found over time that the third option worked wonders for us because my husband is a night owl and I love my sleep! Pick whichever option sounds the most life-giving to the needs of your family and your social life.

OTHER TOPICS
ON THE RADAR

BABY MIXING UP DAYS & NIGHTS

If you find that your baby experiences very little waketime during the day and seems to want to party all night long, he may have his days and nights confused. In the first few months of your baby's life, he is trying to settle into his own circadian rhythm. Some babies naturally align with our rhythms; others need a little assistance. If you are in the latter category, here are some tricks you can implement to get your baby back on a regular day-night routine:

- Wake your baby every 2-3 hours during the day to feed him. You'll need to be structured and diligent with this for several days in order to reverse his cycle.

- Keep your baby awake during his daytime feedings and for a short time afterwards for that "Play" time. This goes back to what we learned in

Chapters 3 and 4 about full feedings and the Eat-Play-Sleep routine. A sleepy baby may be hard to arouse to feed, but it is imperative to squeeze in milk calories during the day so that he isn't relying solely on the nighttime feedings to fill him up. Do what you must to keep that sweet baby awake! Talk to him, tickle his tummy, undress him… I even know moms who have used cold washcloths or ice cubes on their baby's bare feet to keep him awake. Yes, this sounds awful, but keep in mind that this is rooted in the love you have for your baby and your desire to help him find his rhythm and establish a healthy sleep routine.

- Keep natural light around your baby during the day, even when he naps. When surrounded by light, our bodies release a hormone called cortisol, which stimulates alertness. When surrounded by darkness, our bodies release melatonin, which makes us drowsy and signals that it's time for sleep. The catch here is that babies don't start producing melatonin until 6 weeks of age, so some babies will be difficult to "correct" before then. Even so, I recommend staying active during the day, getting your baby exposed to plenty of natural light. This doesn't mean you should put your baby down for naps in a room with all the lights on; it means that you shouldn't go crazy with the blackout curtains and cave-like setting during his daytime naps until he has his days and nights in order.

- During your baby's nighttime wakings, keep the room quiet, calm and dark. Unswaddle your baby during his feeding, change his diaper, then re-swaddle him and put him immediately back to bed. He will most likely resist this initially since he is used to being awake during this time, but remember that this is a learning process and will simply require a little practice and patience before you reach your goal.

EXERCISE FOR MOM

Unless otherwise instructed by your OB, it is safe to start exercising around 4 to 6 weeks postpartum. I highly recommend this for physical and mental health and to practice being away from your baby. I vividly remember the first time I went to the gym by myself after my first son was born. The two of us had become so attached that it felt awkward to be away from him, but I was so glad I started this practice early. This gave my husband a chance for some one-on-one time with our baby, it gave me some space to clear my head, and it inspired me to eat healthier and make strides toward losing my baby weight and feeling like myself again. As with any other discipline in life, this may not feel easy, but it will pay off in your overall well-being.

Take caution in the beginning and try not to overdo it. If you exert yourself too hard, you will notice an increase in your vaginal bleeding and this indicates that you may need to slow down a little. For the first six weeks, skip any exercises that cause your belly to bulge outward, like sit-ups, crunches, or plank. Exercises like these can put extra strain on your midline and actually worsen your post-belly pooch (diastasis recti). Exercises that are generally encouraged for reestablishing core strength are: pelvic tilts, heel slides, oblique curls, and bridges. Check with your OB, have him or her check the status of your abdominal separation, and reincorporate exercises slowly and as you feel ready.

NORMAL DEVELOPMENT: 1 MONTH

- Your baby sees in black and white. He sees bold patterns and notices faces.

- Your baby will start cooing and making some of the most adorable noises you've ever heard.

- Your baby may develop a skin rash on his face, scalp, chest or back. This can be baby acne (small red bumps), milia (tiny white bumps), or pink splotchy areas (drool rash). These are all normal and typically resolve on their own.

- Always lay your baby down to sleep on his back.

- Practice tummy time every day. Lay your baby down on his tummy while he is awake and monitored so he can strengthen his arm and neck muscles. Your baby will probably hate this at first and that is normal. Start with just a few minutes and work towards 5 minutes at a time. He should be able to move his head from side to side.

- Your baby will sleep 16 to 18 hours a day, including nap times.

- Your baby should average 8 to 10 feedings in a 24-hour period.[1]

- Expect 5-8 wet diapers and 3-4 stools daily for the first month.[2] After the first month, the stooling pattern may change and your baby may now pass only one large stool per day or as infrequently as one in every three to five days.[3] Awesome!

- 8 -

WEEK FIVE

PRIMARY FOCUS:
Start a bedtime routine.

Bedtime routines are important for soothing your baby and preparing him for sleep, but let's not get too crazy here. I have seen plenty of parents establish an elaborate bedtime routine that ends up lasting well over an hour, leaving everyone fatigued and burdened in the end. I believe this process should be roughly 20-30 minutes and include things you enjoy and can consistently offer your baby every night. I don't even recommend having bath time as part of the bedtime routine because then you get stuck having to bathe your child EVERY night, and this simply isn't necessary. A bedtime routine should be simple, calming and enjoyable. It should *start* with the baby's last feeding so that you reinforce the separation between feeding and sleep. Next, you will want to include things like: reading a book, singing a song, brushing teeth (when they come in), swaddling (until three months of age) and some soothing cuddles. This routine provides important cues that signal to your baby that it is time for bed. Then you can stay ahead of the meltdown, lay your baby down on his back (drowsy but still awake), and walk out.

Note: I am against the idea of trying to "trick" our babies into falling asleep by laying them down and then sneaking out of the room. We don't want them to wake up feeling confused and betrayed; we want them to know exactly where they are and how they got there. Bedtime should be light-hearted and fun, not associated with any negativity or dread. Babies pick up on our demeanors more than we realize! Be confident and firm when it comes to your baby's sleep routines and cherish this as a time to bond with your baby and gift him with rest.

A consistent bedtime routine has been found to be a predictor of better sleep and fewer night wakings.[1] As your baby gets older, staying firm on bedtime boundaries will become even more important. Yes, it's hard to say no when Little Johnny wants "just one more book" but committing to your limitations reinforces your authority. I learned early on with my kids that "last one" was an important phrase and only remained powerful if I stayed true to it. At one, three, and five years of age, my boys all know that bedtime includes two books, one song, hugs and kisses, and a prayer. THE END. No budging here or I could literally get sucked in for hours! I love spending time with my kids but, in these situations, maintaining my authority and prioritizing their sleep are the appropriate ways to provide for them.

ANOTHER TOPIC ON THE RADAR

MOVING BABY OUT OF YOUR ROOM

When and how to move your baby out of your room is another personal and debated subject, and plenty of moms struggle with this decision. For some, their anxiety increases if the baby is at bedside and Mom wakes up with every little noise the baby makes. For others, the thought of having their baby down the hall or on another floor of the house is what increases their anxiety.

It is worth mentioning that The AAP recommends

keeping a baby in his parent's room until at least six months of age and ideally for one year.[2] Honestly, when I heard this recommendation, I couldn't even imagine it. I am a light sleeper and found myself waking constantly throughout the night with every tiny noise my baby made. My sleep deprivation was increasing my anxiety and even gave me negative feelings toward my baby when his noises would awaken me.

For me, I weighed the options and closely considered all of the risks and benefits involved (see "SIDS Prevention" in Chapter 2). I was cautious with all other recommendations regarding risk factors for SIDS and took into account that my ability to sleep improved my well-being, decreased my stress levels, and helped me be a more attentive and loving mother. Additionally, upon doing more research, I found that a large percentage of infants who die of SIDS are found with their head covered by bedding.[3] Therefore, by following the recommendation to keep my baby's crib free of any blankets, bumpers, lovies, etc., my anxiety decreased tremendously and I felt confident about moving our baby to his own room. We made the choice around this 5-week mark and it was the right decision for our family.

Once our baby started sleeping in his own room, it also helped me delay my response to his cries in the middle of the night, and I believe this enabled him to learn self-soothing techniques much sooner. Sometimes I would wait a few minutes to check on him and by the time I got down to his room he had already soothed himself back to sleep! You will find out in no time that it's extremely difficult to let your baby cry in the middle of the night when he is in your room, screaming *right next to your head*. Every minute your baby cries will feel excruciating and the "quick fix" is to feed him, even though this may not actually be what he needs.

> **Note:** If your partner is a working man, he may really benefit from having your baby out of your room. Assuming you have some time off from work to be home with your baby, you may find that you can sacrifice a walk down the hall to feed him so that you can aid your partner in gaining some extra, uninterrupted sleep.

Consult with your partner and pediatrician and make a plan that fits you and your family's needs.

WEEK SIX

PRIMARY FOCUS:

Establish a first feeding of the day.

It's important to establish a first feeding of the day if you want your baby's schedule to look consistent from day to day. This means that you decide when you want each day to start and you set this as your baby's daily alarm clock (ideally within a ½ hour range each day). Establishing consistency in your baby's routine will help to stabilize his metabolism and his sleep-wake cycles.[1] Additional research shows that this simple change can dramatically reduce night wakings.[2] Need I say more?

- Example: If you choose your baby's first feeding time to be at 7am, some days you will feed your baby closer to 6:30am if he wakes up early, or you will wake him up and feed him closer to 7:30am if he sleeps in.

- o For this example, feedings on a 3-hour routine would occur at (roughly) 7am, 10am, 1pm, 4pm, 7pm, 10pm, 1am, and 4am (see sample schedule).

- o For the late evening feeding (10pm), treat this as bedtime and implement your bedtime routine. You are nearing the phase when you can drop that late evening feeding and start putting your baby to bed around 8pm.

Note: If you are a working mom on maternity leave, you may wish to temporarily set this first feeding at a later hour and slowly move it forward when the time comes to return to work. No need for a 6am wakeup time when you're on "vacation," am I right? For example, I set my baby's first feeding at 8am initially and then slowly cut it back by 15-minute increments until I reached the 6:30am wakeup time we would need when I returned to work. This shifted his entire schedule earlier but, by doing it slowly, this was virtually unnoticed by my baby.

At this point, your baby's schedule should range from 2 ½- to 3 ½-hour intervals with 8 to 10 feedings per day (or 7-8 feedings per day once he is sleeping through the night). Around 8 to 10 weeks, your baby will drop the early morning feeding(s) and can sleep 7 to 8 hours, so this is a great thing to keep in mind when these nights start to feel really long!

Sample Schedule (3-hour routine)

7:00am	Wake baby for first feeding, diaper change, play/awake time, nap
10:00am	Feeding, diaper change, play/awake time, nap
1:00pm	Feeding, diaper change, play/awake time, nap
4:00pm	Feeding, diaper change, play/awake time, nap
7:00pm	Feeding, diaper change, play/awake time, nap
10:00pm	Feeding, diaper change, bedtime routine, down for the night
During the Night	Feeding, diaper change, re-swaddle, then immediately back down for the

(1-3 times)	night

TROUBLESHOOTING

What if you have established your "first feeding" at 7am but your baby wakes up crying at 5am? You have two choices: 1) You can let your baby cry for a bit and see if he falls back to sleep on his own, or 2) You can feed your baby at 5am, put him immediately back down to sleep (treating this as if it is still nighttime), then wake him again at 7/7:30am to feed him and start your day. He may not take a full feeding at this time, but you can still start his Eat-Play-Sleep routine and keep him on his consistent daily rhythm.

ANOTHER TOPIC ON THE RADAR

SEX AFER BABY

Let's talk about sex, baby. I know, I know… but before you roll your eyes at me and throw this book across the room, hear me out. Sex is an important part of any relationship and the thing that got us here in the first place, so I believe it deserves to be acknowledged. Also, chances are this will be your male counterpart's favorite section of this book. Since he's endured talk on nipples and colostrum, I think he deserves a break.

For starters, let's reflect back to my beliefs on parenting, assuming you agree with them. This little baby has taken over a lot of the attention and focus of your lives right now, but don't forget that you and your partner and the health of your relationship takes priority. I know you're tired and perhaps a little edgy and irritable, but the intimacy of your relationship still deserves attention. Your OB will generally give you the go-ahead for sex around 6 weeks postpartum, but the decision to reintroduce this is completely up to you and your partner.

> **Note:** Remember that hormone, oxytocin, that we talked about with breastfeeding? Don't be alarmed when it is stimulated during sex and causes the let-down reflex to release some milk from your breasts. Try to laugh about it, wear a bra during sex if it bothers you, and know that it's all part of this fun, wild ride!

- **To the Fellas:** Try a little tenderness. Don't forget that your sweet lady just went through the most insane physical and emotional transition known to mankind. She's getting used to her new body, to skin that sags where it didn't used to, to cellulite in new places, to boobs that feel like they belong to someone else. Be gentle and encouraging towards her, continue to pursue her, and remind her how much you love her and find her attractive. Think outside the box for ways to tend to her right now: fill up her water bottle while she's nursing... give her a back rub while you're watching a movie... plan a date night out of the house... when in doubt, buy chocolate!

- **To the Ladies:** It is totally normal to have some fear and apprehension about sex after childbirth. For some, it is painful and awkward physically; for others, it is surprisingly enjoyable and welcome. Don't be afraid to talk openly with your partner about what feels good and what doesn't. He has hopefully shown patience and respect during this time, but a sure way to love him is to at least attempt to acknowledge this topic and his physical needs. Also, give yourself some grace. No, your body will not look like it did when you were a teenager, but don't forget that you just delivered a live HUMAN BEING. How incredible! You are a rock star!

Note: Always use protection! The myth that breastfeeding is a good contraceptive has been widely debunked. Just ask my friend who had babies 11 months apart!

WEEK SEVEN

PRIMARY FOCUS:

Maintain your sanity.

Okay sisters, here's the thing: This period has always been hard for me. At this point you are sleep-deprived, covered in milk, irritable towards your partner, and the shine of your sweet, little one has somewhat worn off. You may be asking yourself questions like: *Did I make a mistake? Do I even love this baby? Will he ever do anything other than cry and poop? Do I have any idea what I'm doing?* Let me say this clearly: YOU ARE NOT ALONE. You are a good mom, you were made specifically to be *this* baby's mom, and you are doing one heck of a job. Also... THIS WILL GET BETTER.

This period is also notorious for the first of many

growth spurts for your baby and this can wreak havoc on any kind of routine you've created. Just when you thought Little Johnny was finally stretching out his nighttime feedings, he is awake again every 3 hours. Even worse, he is waking up early from his naps too! In this case – and assuming the growth spurt is to blame – you will still want to delay your response to him (try 7 minutes if you're able) and feed him at that point if he is still crying, as this may indicate a true hunger cry. If he takes a full feeding, you will know that the growth spurt is to blame and you can then adjust his next feeding to get back on his routine. This will not mess up his ability to sleep longer stretches. It is simply meeting his current need for more calories. After a few days/nights, he will be right back on track to stretching out his nighttime feedings. Hang in there!

ANOTHER TOPIC ON THE RADAR

POSTPARTUM DEPRESSION & ANXIETY

This is a real thing, my friends. I experienced this after my second son was born and it was fierce, abrupt and oppressive. I am usually a positive, outgoing, happy person, but all of that went out the window without warning. I felt sad in ways I had never known sadness before. I worried about the smallest, most bizarre things. I literally felt crazy at times. I even had thoughts about harming my baby. MY DARLING, SQUISHY BABY. This made no sense to me at the time and I could even recognize how ridiculous it was, yet it still felt very real and scary. I finally swallowed my pride and said something to my husband, then to my OB, then started seeing a counselor who helped me release some of these fears into the world.

What I learned by the time my third baby came around is that babies are more resilient than we realize, and they certainly aren't judging us as harshly as we are judging ourselves. When we hold ourselves to an unattainable standard of perfection, it is a disservice to ourselves and to our babies. It is okay to make mistakes and feel confused or overwhelmed. It is okay if you spilled the bottle or you forgot to change a diaper or you had to let your baby cry for a few minutes while you took a deep breath in the other room. You are not perfect, and you were never meant to be perfect. Embracing that with grace for yourself is the biggest hurdle, but also an incredible gift to model to your baby. Be kind to yourself. Parenthood is a learning process and one that takes practice and patience. Your baby wants you and only you, just the way you are.

If you are experiencing feelings of sadness, loneliness, guilt, shame, fear, regret, anxiety, or especially if you have thoughts of harming yourself or your baby, please GET HELP. If you need to see a counselor, go on medication, and/or figure out a plan to get more rest or alone time, this does not make you a bad mom. This makes you brave and responsible and I am proud of you. This does not mean you don't love your child. It means you are prioritizing your own self-care to *better* love your child.

WEEK EIGHT

PRIMARY FOCUS:
Introduce crying intervals & check-ins.

This is a great time to start letting your baby cry a bit longer at naps and bedtime in order to teach him how to self-soothe and sleep independently. When deciding how much crying to allow, use your discretion and decide on a time interval that feels right to you. Using my rule of thumb, aim for *at least* 8 minutes since he is 8 weeks old. However, keep in mind that this time interval is actually more for your sanity than it is for your baby's well-being. Continue to ask yourself the question: *Is my baby unsafe or is he simply uncomfortable?* While letting your baby cry for longer periods of time may feel harsh, the total amount of crying will be less if you can tolerate longer time intervals from the get-go. If you are comfortable with 30-45 minutes, that is ideal, and you will likely see improvements sooner.

At this stage, I would cuddle my baby and prepare him for sleep, swaddle him tightly, put him down in his crib (while he was still awake but showing signs of drowsiness), set a timer for the decided time interval, then walk out of the room. (I highly recommend setting a timer so that it can hold you accountable to the time interval you have set). Next, I would go hang out with my husband, turn up the tv, or put on some headphones to drown out the noise until the timer went off. You may wish to utilize a video monitor during the crying interval, as this will help to ensure that your baby is simply uncomfortable but is not unsafe.

If the timer goes off, your baby is still crying, and it feels unbearable to listen to him cry any longer (and believe me, I get it!) then you may wish to implement a "check-in." With a check-in, you will go back into your baby's room, rub his tummy, sing a song and offer his pacifier, but I do not recommend picking him up at this point. It is okay to reassure him of your presence and love, but picking him up tends to reset the whole process and lead to *harder* crying. If you do wish to pick up your baby, rock him and soothe him until he is calm, but lay him back down while he is still awake. Then you will set the timer again (ideally for at least 5 minutes longer than the previous time interval) and repeat the process until your baby has soothed himself to sleep. It will be incredibly hard to listen to your baby cry, but try your best to maintain the bigger perspective and the importance of teaching your baby how to sleep independently. Remember: a baby who sleeps well is a gift to the whole family!

As your baby gets older, you will want to lengthen the check-in intervals as you feel comfortable. In this stage of sleep training for a baby who has followed The BSB Method, I have found that these crying spells take roughly three to five nights to overcome and can take more like 1-2 weeks to solidify for nap times. The crying typically lasts an average of 20-45 minutes the first night, about half that amount of time the second night, and only about 10 minutes or less on the third night. Of course, this is not an exact science and every baby will be different. It's helpful to keep in mind that each night will potentially improve upon the night before and your hope of a quiet household throughout the night is now a tangible reality to grasp.

Note: At this stage of your baby's development, I recommend implementing these sleep training strategies for bedtime and naps *simultaneously* so as not to confuse your baby about what is expected of him. Some parents want to get nighttime sleep solidified before implementing sleep training for naps, but this may be confusing for your baby. If you rock or nurse him to sleep for naps *or* bedtime, he is going to expect that *all the time*. Use a consistent method for putting your baby down to sleep: drowsy but awake, alone in his crib.

That being said, if your baby has a particularly fussy day and is fighting his naps, you may find it more soothing to both of you to rock him to sleep for his next nap. That is okay! Consistency is the key, but you aren't going to spoil all your efforts by deviating from the norm from time to time. Don't let any of this produce anxiety in you. You love your baby and you are doing your best to help him… that is the most important thing!

ANOTHER TOPIC
ON THE RADAR

DITCHING THE SWADDLE

Most experts agree that swaddling should be discontinued around 2-3 months of age, or when your baby starts to roll over.[1] It is normal for your baby to protest this a bit, just as he would with any change in his comfort level. Keep in mind that removing a swaddle is not harming him. It may take several days/nights of consistency before you can expect him to give in without a fight. Try one arm out for 3 nights, then both arms out for 3 nights, then remove the swaddle altogether.

NORMAL DEVELOPMENT: 2 MONTHS

- Your baby will start to smile at you (and this is the best thing ever!).

- Your baby will start tracking with his eyes, following objects and recognizing people at a distance.

- Continue practicing tummy time every day. Lay your baby down on his tummy while he is awake and monitored so he can strengthen his arm and neck muscles. He may begin to push up and hold his head up. He may still cry and fuss over this, but it's important! Work towards 5 minutes at a time and increase as your baby can tolerate it.

- Crying is normal and may increase around this time as your baby is awake for longer stretches during the day.[1]

- Your baby may start to roll over, so be extremely cautious about leaving him on high surfaces unattended.

- You may start giving Tylenol at 2 months of age (but no Ibuprofen/Motrin until 6 months).

> **BOSS tip:** When giving medication to a baby, use a syringe and squirt slowly into the pocket of his cheek. If he protests or holds his breath, hold him firmly and blow in his face, as this will force him to swallow.

- Feed your baby 6-8 times each day.

- Healthy, full-term babies can sleep 7-9 hours continuously at this point. If your baby is continuing to feed every 3 hours during the night, consider letting him cry longer before responding for a feeding, knowing in confidence that he does not *need* this feeding but is simply expecting it based on habit.

- Ideas for Play: reading, play gym, singing, going for a walk outside.

- 13 -

WEEKS NINE TO TWELVE

PRIMARY FOCUS:
Transition back to work.

If you are a working mom, your maternity leave may be coming to an end soon (if it hasn't already). It is totally okay and normal to have mixed emotions about this. With each of my babies, I felt an incredible sense of sadness and loss about the ending of maternity leave (even dramatically proclaiming "It's the end of an ERA!"), but I also felt some excitement and anticipation about returning to work. Hopefully at this point you have become well-acquainted with your breast pump, but you will now have the added challenge of taking this to work and implementing this into your new routine. I won't lie, this is hard at times, but I am proud of you for sticking with it!

Upon returning to work, your baby may be entering a new setting at daycare, in-home care, or care from a nanny or family member. A lot of moms experience anxiety at this time, wondering if and how their baby's schedule will be maintained in this new setting. While I do believe it can be helpful to offer your baby's schedule to his new caregiver, I hope you will understand that this can't always be followed to a tee. My word of encouragement from experience and research is this: your baby will be fine. Because you have raised your baby to be adaptable, he will show off his flexibility skills and adjust to his new surroundings. When back at home, he will adjust back to his home routine. While it is definitely hard to leave your baby in someone else's care, I truly believe you will see the benefit of surrendering control. Keep in mind that the most important thing is not that your baby's routine is followed perfectly but that he is safe and loved.

If you find that your baby is particularly fussy after a day with a caregiver, put him to bed at an earlier hour that night to prevent him from getting overtired. Stay ahead of the meltdown!

ANOTHER TOPIC
ON THE RADAR

STOPPING THE MIDDLE-OF-THE-NIGHT DIAPER CHANGES

That's right, unless your baby is poopy, you can now skip this step and make the nighttime wakings less of an event. Feed your baby during the night when he is (truly) hungry, burp him, then immediately put him back down. Hopefully this is only happening once during the night at this point (if at all).

THREE TO FIVE MONTHS

PRIMARY FOCUS:

Drop the Late PM feeding and put your baby to bed earlier (around 8pm).

Your baby should now have 4-6 feedings during the day and can extend nighttime sleep to 9-11 hours. HECK. YES. Assuming your baby is in good health and this is approved by his pediatrician, by the time he is three months old and weighs at least 13 pounds he is fully capable of sleeping through the night without a feeding (insert angels singing).[1]

Some parents are surprised by the idea of putting their baby to bed *earlier* for fear that he will now wake up at an earlier hour in the morning. Conversely, studies have shown that a baby will wake up at a consistent time each day no matter what time he has gone to bed at night.[2] Additionally, earlier bedtimes help prevent bedtime battles, deter night waking, and prolong naptimes during the day.[3] Therefore, putting your baby to bed at an earlier hour will give him a longer stretch of nighttime sleep, which will benefit the entire family.

Another huge benefit of this earlier bedtime for your baby is much-needed alone time with your partner. My husband and I absolutely love when our boys go to bed at night and we have found that this time we have together is invaluable to the health of our relationship. We can catch up on our days, watch a movie, or have friends over, all without the interruption of a baby. You might find that you struggle with this initially, just as I did. After spending a day away at work, I would often long for time with my baby and miss him as soon as I put him to bed. This is normal, but it doesn't mean you should compromise this time that is so vital to your baby's development and to your relationship with your partner.

By three to five months of age, your baby can be on a consistent routine with three naps a day, each lasting roughly 1 to 2 hours. Keep in mind that all babies are different; some will sleep longer, some won't nap as long, and some may only want two naps. The most important indicator of rest is a content and happy baby.

Even though the most high-quality sleep will occur at home in the crib, let's be realistic regarding your sanity and social life. My aim was always to get at least *one* solid nap at home, whereas the other 1-2 would take place on-the-go in a stroller or car seat. This benefited my mental well-being by getting me time out of the house with my girl friends, and made me a happier, more-attentive mom. If I could foresee that his nap was going to conflict with one of my social events, I would put him down to sleep in his car seat (in his room) and then quietly transfer him to the car when it was time to leave.

Here is a sample schedule of what an average day might look like. Keep in mind that the timeline can be adjusted according to you and your baby's routine.

Sample Schedule: 3-5 Months
(3 Naps)

7:00am	Wake baby for first feeding, diaper change, play/awake time
9:00am	Nap (1 ½ - 2 hours)
10:30/11am	Baby wakes up, feeding, diaper change, play/awake time
1:00pm	Nap (1 ½ - 2 hours)
2:30pm	Baby wakes up, feeding, diaper change, play/awake time
4:00pm	Nap (1 - 2 hours)
5/5:30pm	Baby wakes up, feeding, diaper change, play/awake time
7:30pm	Feeding (This is the only feeding that will occur sooner than the 3-4-hour range but will ensure your baby has a full tummy before bedtime), diaper change, pj's, bedtime routine
8/8:30pm	Bedtime

Note: Keep in mind that when it says "Baby wakes

up," this will be a rough estimate of when your baby will naturally wake up from his nap on his own. If your baby naps for longer than 2 ½ hours during the day, I suggest waking him up for his feeding so that he maintains his rhythm and still relies on the nighttime for that longer stretch of sleep.

Note: If your baby is still waking once or twice during the night to feed (and isn't having issues with weight gain), consider letting him cry for longer stretches until he soothes himself back to sleep. Some babies may still need one night feeding until around six months of age, but the majority can go without.

ANOTHER TOPIC
ON THE RADAR

TEETHING

Most babies cut their first tooth around 4 to 7 months of age, although this can vary drastically from baby to baby. Signs of teething include: drooling, irritability, swollen gums, rosy cheeks, low-grade fevers, trouble sleeping and loose stools. Sounds fun, doesn't it?

Once that first tooth pops through, you've got a few

things to think about:

1. *How adorable is my baby right now?!* The two-bottom-teeth phase is seriously the cutest!

2. Watch out, breastfeeding moms! Teething babies are in search of anything and everything they can gnaw on and unfortunately this might include your nipple at times - ouch! It is okay to give your baby a gentle flick on the cheek and firmly tell him "No" when he bites you.

3. You can start brushing that tiny tooth with a soft bristle toothbrush with water or even just wiping it with a wet washcloth once or twice a day to prevent tooth decay.

4. *What can I do to stop this madness?* Care for a teething baby is another subject of debate and controversy. Some parents swear by amber teething necklaces and homeopathic treatments; others opt for teething gels, teething toys, and good, old-fashioned Tylenol. Do your research and choose an approach that matches your convictions and goals.

> **BOSS tip:** Once your baby can grasp an object, you can put a wet washcloth in the freezer and

then give it to your baby to chew on.

- 15 -

NORMAL DEVELOPMENT:
6 MONTHS

- Your baby should be able to sit unaided.

- Your baby can pass items from one hand to the other.

- Some babies start crawling around six months of age so it's a good time to think about child-proofing your home. This includes covering electrical outlets, clearing the area of small objects, placing child-proof gadgets on kitchen and bathroom drawers and lower cabinets, and placing baby gates at the top and/or bottom of stairways.

- Your baby will start making sounds and you can encourage communication by copying the sounds he makes. Yes, you will look ridiculous, but who cares?! Your baby thinks you are the coolest thing since the Diaper Genie®!

- Believe it or not, your baby can understand simple words by now. If you are planning to use Baby Sign Language, this is a good time to start introducing some simple signs like "more," "all done," "milk," and "please."

- Most babies will have doubled their birth weight and growth will start to slow down.

- You may now give Ibuprofen as needed for the occasional teething symptoms or fever.

- Your baby can eat solid foods 2-3 times a day (see Chapter 16 for more details on this).[1]

- Ideas for Play: patty-cake, peek-a-boo, board books, looking in a mirror.

SIX TO NINE MONTHS

PRIMARY FOCUS:
Introduce solid foods.

Solid foods can be introduced to your baby as early as four months, but I don't recommend this unless your baby is showing an obvious interest in food. Starting solids can be a fun process, but it is also messy, time-consuming and, honestly, a little annoying at times, especially since you've developed a smooth feeding schedule by now. Here are some recommendations on what to start with:

- The AAP recommends introducing new foods one at a time. A great introductory food is an iron-fortified cereal mixed with breastmilk or formula.

- Introduce pureed fruits and vegetables. Offer 1-2 tablespoons of pureed food twice a day, then work towards three times a day (see sample schedules provided). Keep in mind that the majority of your baby's nutrients are provided through breastmilk or formula until 12 months of age, so don't worry about how much food your baby is taking in. This is all just a fun learning process!

> **Note:** When introducing pureed fruits and vegetables from a jar or pouch, empty a couple of tablespoons into a separate container to feed your baby from. The bacteria in a baby's mouth can contaminate the jar (via the spoon) and would need to be thrown out. An uncontaminated jar or pouch can be refrigerated and used within 48 hours of opening.

- Research from The AAP suggests that early introduction of highly allergenic foods may prevent food allergies from developing.[1] Around 6 to 9 months, your baby's immune system is maturing and can create antigens to combat these allergens, so this is a good time frame to introduce these foods to your baby. This includes: dairy, eggs, peanuts, tree nuts, fish, shellfish, soy and wheat.

> **BOSS tip:** When introducing peanut butter, add a teaspoon of *powdered* peanut butter to your baby's rice cereal. This exposes him to peanuts without posing a choking risk.

- Foods to avoid: raw honey (can cause botulism and should be avoided until one year of age), large or hard chunks of food that your baby could choke on, i.e. raisins, nuts, popcorn, hot dogs, and raw vegetables.

Note: After starting solids, many babies experience constipation as their bodies learn to adjust and digest these new foods. If your baby is having hard, pebble-like stools and/or crying out in pain during bowel movements, avoid bananas, rice, and carrots, which can contribute to constipation. Instead, once or twice a day, add one of "The 6 P's" to his diet, which each help to soften the stools and relieve constipation.

The 6 P's: prunes, pears, pumpkin, plums, peaches, and peas.

If your baby does not experience relief, and especially if he has persistent vomiting, abdominal tenderness, or a decreased appetite, notify your pediatrician as soon as possible.

Once your child is sitting up and taking pureed foods well, it's time to start finger foods. Great options for finger foods include: cubed avocado, Cheerios, yogurt melts, puffed cereal, diced bananas, and soft meats. Additionally, I recommend offering your baby anything you are eating that piques his interest (that isn't a choking hazard, of course!). Babies who are only offered "kid foods" will continue to want these types of options. If you offer your baby things like quinoa, guacamole, beans, scrambled eggs, soft cheeses, etc., you may be surprised how diverse his palate will become!

BOSS tip: While I recommend offering fruits and vegetables in their whole forms, it can also be beneficial to "hide" them in foods to increase your child's intake. For example, in our house of boys we have green "Hulk Mac-n-Cheese" and "Hulk Pancakes," both of which have pureed spinach added to the liquid base. While this may sound disgusting, I promise you can't taste it! You can also hide tons of vegetables into soups or stews by pureeing them into the broth.

ANOTHER TOPIC
ON THE RADAR

DROPPING A NAP

At this stage your baby should average 3-4 hours of total daytime sleep and may be ready to drop the late afternoon nap.

Making a change in your baby's schedule can be anxiety-producing and daunting. After all, you've finally settled into a routine that works for you and your busy life! First and foremost, you want to observe your baby and follow his cues on whether or not he is needing all three naps. Of course, there is no perfect science to a nap schedule, but if your baby is having more trouble falling asleep for naps or napping for shorter periods, he may be ready to drop a nap.

- The easiest way I have found to do this is by deciding off the bat what the ideal timing for those two naps would be. For me, those times were around 9am and 2pm. Because my baby was used to taking that afternoon nap earlier (because it was his second of *three* naps) I found that being on the go and doing something stimulating during that time helped to distract him and keep him awake in order to stretch out the time between naps. Simply put: no driving in a car or taking a walk in the stroller while we were in transition times because those are his typical sleep triggers. At the time he was previously starting his second nap (around 12:30pm), I would read him a book, stack blocks with him, or do anything else that would distract him and keep him stimulated. After a little while, he would start to show signs of drowsiness, so I would change his diaper and prepare him for naptime.

- When it comes time to actually drop that third nap, I would suggest implementing your ideal schedule and sticking to it. Because you have raised your baby to be adaptable, he will eventually adjust accordingly. Remember, consistently follow a structured routine in order to create flexibility! *Will this go smoothly right away?* Probably not. Give it 3-5 days of consistent efforts and watch in amazement as your sweet, little one takes his next step towards independence and growth.

- I would advise against dropping a nap around holidays or travel, as these situations can naturally disrupt his sleep patterns.

- It is also important to remember that your baby is a human being and not a robot. Even as an adult, most days I feel energized and alert; some days I feel sluggish and need a nap. Your baby will be the same and that is okay. He may transition smoothly down to two naps but still need an occasional late afternoon cat nap from time to time.

Now that you have dropped down to two naps and added solids into your baby's routine, you can start putting your baby to bed at a time that should remain consistent for the next several years of his life (around 7-7:30pm). Remember that the goal should be to get your baby down for the night while he is drowsy but before he is overtired. Some babies reach this window even earlier (around 6-6:30pm), especially if they've had an exhausting day at daycare. Observe your baby and get him to bed during that window to prevent protesting at bedtime. Stay ahead of the meltdown!

Here is a sample schedule of what a typical day might look like:

Sample Schedule: 6-9 Months
(2 Naps + 2 Solids)

6:30/7am	Wake baby for first feeding, diaper change, play/awake time
8:00am	Solids
9:00am	Nap (1 ½ - 2 hours)
11:00am	Baby wakes up, feeding, diaper change, play/awake time
1:30/2pm	Nap (1 ½ - 2 hours)
4:00pm	Baby wakes up, feeding, diaper change, play/awake time
5:00pm	Solids
6:30/7pm	Feeding, diaper change, pj's, bedtime routine
7/7:30pm	Bedtime

Note: Keep in mind that when it says "Baby wakes up," this will be a rough estimate of when your baby will naturally wake up from his nap on his own. If your baby naps for longer than 3 hours during the day, I suggest waking him up for his feeding so that he maintains his rhythm and still relies on the nighttime for that longer stretch of sleep.

- 17 -

NORMAL DEVELOPMENT: 9 MONTHS

- Your baby should make a variety of sounds, like "mamama" and "dadada."

- Talk to your baby as if he understands what you're saying. Tell him "It's time to eat" or "It's time to go night-night."

- Use "No!" only when your baby is going to get hurt or could hurt others.[1]

- Your baby may start to point at things that pique his interest.

- Your baby should be crawling and may even start "furniture surfing," so child-proofing your home is a must. This includes covering electrical outlets, clearing the area of small objects, placing child-proof gadgets on kitchen and bathroom drawers

123

and lower cabinets, and placing baby gates at the top and/or bottom of stairways.

- Offer finger foods that are soft, small and healthy. A baby can try something 10-12 times before liking it and this is as frustrating as it sounds. Some babies are experimental eaters and some won't eat anything even remotely healthy, but I have found that it is beneficial to consistently *try*. Model good eating behaviors and offer healthy options first when your baby is most hungry.

- Your baby can start using a cup to drink from (with your help). This will be messy, but it's super cute!

- Your baby may start to cry and show distress when you leave him and this is a normal phase called "Separation Anxiety." This doesn't mean you should never leave your baby's side; usually a baby can be distracted and redirected within minutes. It is important for your baby to see you come and go to establish trust and independence. Did someone say, "Happy Hour"?

- Ideas for Play: balls, toys that stack and roll, blocks, containers.

TEN TO TWELVE MONTHS

PRIMARY FOCUS:

Transition to a sippy or straw cup.

Some babies can transition to a sippy or straw cup as early as six months and some don't show interest until twelve months, so don't let yourself get too stressed out if this doesn't come naturally to your baby. All of my babies preferred a straw cup over the traditional sippy cup but couldn't get down the sucking ability until around ten months of age. There are some great YouTube videos that demonstrate ways to teach your baby how to drink from a straw cup, so I won't explain this in detail.

Once your baby is drinking successfully from a straw or sippy cup, you can replace one of his bottle- or breastfeeding sessions by offering breastmilk or formula in his cup of choice. This will also help if you're hoping to wean your baby from breastfeeding around his first birthday (see more below).

ANOTHER TOPIC ON THE RADAR

WEANING

The decision to wean your baby from breastfeeding can come with a mixed bag of emotions. Part of you might want to rewind time and do it all over again; another part of you may be getting excited about the prospect of new independence and freedom for yourself. There is no perfect science about when and how to wean your baby, but since The AAP recommends breastfeeding until one year of age, that is a great goal to strive for. There are also a variety of strategies on *how* to wean your baby, but I will describe in detail what worked for me.

- It is best to wean your baby by first implementing the change to one of his afternoon feedings since this is naturally when your milk supply will be lower. Simply give your baby a bottle (or cup of choice) with breastmilk or formula and don't pump at that time.

- If you are a working mom and were accustomed to pumping twice during the day, aim to pump once instead, ideally at a time that is somewhat in between the previous two sessions. For example, if you were used to pumping at 10am and 2pm, aim to pump once at 12pm. I always found that I could go roughly 6-7 hours until the next feeding before feeling uncomfortably full.

- If you become uncomfortably full before his next feeding, you can "pump to comfort" (just for a few minutes), but *do not empty your breasts completely* as this will stimulate more milk production and backtrack your progress. Continue this routine for the next week or so to allow your body to adjust accordingly.

- Next, do the same thing with any of his other daytime feedings until you are only nursing your baby first thing in the morning and last thing at night. This is my absolute favorite period of breastfeeding and I always like to prolong this for my own peace and comfort, and as a way of cherishing the ending of this season. You can make this last as long as you want and/or your body allows.

- Next, cut out that last PM feeding before bedtime. At this time, you can offer your baby a bottle (or cup of choice) at the time you would normally nurse him, then implement your bedtime routine and put him down for the night.

- Lastly, stop nursing him in the morning. This is the hardest feeding for me to cut, and it honestly felt weird to give my baby a straw cup when he first woke up, but by then he was twelve months old and fully capable of surviving life without me (Waaaah!). He may resist this for a while and need to be bottle-fed by your partner, but I promise he will be okay and so will you.

- It always takes me about two weeks of "grieving" before I feel good about being done with breastfeeding. Then – out of the blue – it's like a switch goes off and I feel like a new woman. Breakfast dates with my man! Girls' weekends away! The sky is the limit!

- I have always found it helpful to plan some sort of celebration for myself to help me reach my weaning goals. After baby number one, this was a trip to Mexico with my husband. After baby number two, it was a solo day in the mountains, no babies or breast pumps in sight! It is a bittersweet period but a huge accomplishment to be celebrated, no matter how long you were able to breastfeed.

> **BOSS tip:** At 12 months of age, you can start giving your baby a bottle with whole milk. Some babies protest this initially, so you may wish to start this transition by offering a bottle with one-third whole milk and two-thirds breastmilk, then slowly increasing the ratio of whole milk until your baby takes it without a fuss.

Now that your baby can add more solids to his routine, here is a sample schedule of what a typical day might look like:

Sample Schedule: 10-12 Months
(2 Naps + 3 Meals)

6:30/7am	Wake baby for first feeding, diaper change, play/awake time

8:00am	Breakfast
8:30/9am	Nap (1 ½ - 2 hours)
10:30am	Baby wakes up, feeding, diaper change, play/awake time
12:00pm	Lunch
1:30/2pm	Nap (1 ½ - 2 hours)
4:00pm	Baby wakes up, feeding, diaper change, play/awake time
5/5:30pm	Dinner
6:30pm	Feeding, diaper change, pj's, bedtime routine
7/7:30pm	Bedtime

Note: Keep in mind that when it says "Baby wakes up," this will be a rough estimate of when your baby will naturally wake up from his nap on his own. If your baby naps for longer than 3 hours during the day, I suggest waking him up for his feeding so that he maintains his rhythm and still relies on the nighttime for that longer stretch of sleep.

19

NORMAL DEVELOPMENT: 12 MONTHS

- Your baby can respond to simple spoken directions and requests.

- He can start to use basic gestures, like waving "bye-bye" or shaking his head "no."

- Your baby can say "mama" and "dada" and simple exclamations like "uh-oh!"

- Your baby may stand alone, cruise along furniture, or even take his first steps!

- Encourage your baby to feed himself. Offer a small spoon or fork at mealtimes. He can now add a few things to his menu: honey and cow's milk. Party!

- Fear of strangers is normal and peaks at age one.[1]

- Use short timeouts when your child starts misbehaving. A good rule of thumb is 1 minute per year of age, so a 1-minute timeout is sufficient at this point.

- Brush your baby's teeth twice a day with a soft toothbrush. Use a small smear of fluoride toothpaste (the size of a grain of rice).

- The first-year molars start popping through around 13-19 months, so be on the lookout for some fun signs of teething.

- Schedule your baby for his first visit to the dentist if you haven't already. Most dental offices offer free visits until two years of age and it's nice to get your baby acquainted with this setting.

- Start family traditions for holidays and/or special events. I absolutely love seeing all the creative ways families have captured their children's personalities over the years and around your child's first birthday is a great time to start.

20

CLOSING

Well, you did it! You may be reading this book in its entirety before the arrival of your sweet baby or maybe you're celebrating his first birthday right now. Either way, I am so proud of you. No matter which concepts you decided to adopt or ditch from this book, you did the hard work of seeking knowledge and making informed decisions on how to raise your baby, and that is no small feat!

My hope is that you are left feeling confident, empowered and rested. That you and your partner are still laughing and smiling together, making time for each other, and enjoying parenthood together. That your baby is sleeping through the night, feeling loved, secure and nurtured. That you can share your knowledge and model to other parents what it looks like to thrive in parenthood, not just survive.

Congratulations! You are officially The Next Baby Sleep Boss.

- 21 -

ACKNOWLEDGMENTS

I feel forever indebted to so many wonderful friends and family members who contributed thoughts and ideas for this book.

First and foremost, thank you to Jesus, the kindest friend and wisest teacher of all. You gave me a heart to love, a passion to write, and a more adventurous journey than I could have ever dreamed.

Thank you to my mom, Penny Brown, and my mother-in-law, Joy Fontenot, who both read and edited the book in its beginning stages and were gracious with their feedback. Thank you to Caroline Fontenot, Sarah Hook, Amy Fletcher, Kristen Kramer, Karina Crouch, Lindsay Keller, Anna Siliciano, Katie Layton, Mallory Farokhmanesh, Nancy Daharsh, Katie Everett, Mackenzie Matthews, Lindsey Locker, Amy Callaway, Katy Pfiffner, and countless other sister friends who provided the encouragement I needed to see this to fruition. Thank you to Scott and Abbie Kempin, Ashley and Kara Dreyfuss, and Davin and Holly Lindwall, who were the first couples to trial these concepts and provide insightful feedback along the way.

Thank you to my three boys – Kepler, Crew, and Lincoln – for happily watching more shows than usual during this writing process, for forgiving me when I missed your question the first six times, and, most importantly, for being the amazing and adaptable sleepers that inspired these concepts to come to life in the first place. I love you bigger than the universe and all of its galaxies.

I owe my ability to write this book to my wonderful husband and teammate, Michael. Your positivity and grace toward me in this process have been nothing short of admirable. You listened patiently as I constantly bounced around ideas and dreams surrounding this project, and you cheered me on every step of the way. Thank you for believing in me and for providing the kind of partnership I now have the passion to inspire others toward. I still can't believe this is the life we get to live together.

Last but not least, I'd like to thank YOU, sweet parents. I've said it before and I'll say it again… I am so proud of you for taking the time to educate yourself to better care for your baby. May your hard work and dedication pay off with long nights of sleep and a happy, thriving home.

22

REFERENCES

INTRODUCTION
1. Callahan, A. (2015). PDX Parent: The Science of Sleep. Retrieved from https://www.pdxparent.com/the-science-of-sleep-jan16/
2. Obleman, D. (2007). *The Sleep Sense Program: Proven Strategies For Teaching Your Child To Sleep Through The Night*, p. 13.
3. Ezzo, G. & Bucknam, R. (2006). *On Becoming Babywise: Giving Your Infant the Gift of Nighttime Sleep (4th edition)*, p. 54.

CHAPTER 2: HOT TOPICS FOR NEW PARENTS
1. Centers for Disease Control and Prevention. (2018). About 3,500 babies in the US are lost to sleep-related deaths each year. Retrieved from https://www.cdc.gov/media/releases/2018/p0109-sleep-related-deaths.html.
2. Weissbluth, M. (2015). *Healthy Sleep Habits, Happy Child (Fourth edition)*, p. 137.
3. Weissbluth, M. (2015). *Healthy Sleep Habits, Happy Child (Fourth edition)*, p. 60.
4. What to Expect. (2015). Should you give your baby a pacifier? Retrieved from

https://www.whattoexpect.com/baby-products/pacifiers/.

5. Aldrich, C. A., Sung, C., and Knop, C. (1945). The crying of newly born babies. III. The early period at home. *Journal of Pediatrics*, p. 27, 428-435.

6. USA Today. (2016). Study: Letting a baby cry-it-out won't cause damage. Retrieved from https://www.usatoday.com/story/news/nation-now/2016/05/24/study-infant-baby-sleep-method-cry-it-out-wont-damage-child/84838958/.

7. Duke Department of Pediatrics. (2017). Sleep training your child: myths and facts every parent should know. Retrieved from https://pediatrics.duke.edu/news/sleep-training-your-child-myths-and-facts-every-parent-should-know

8. Obleman, D. (2007). *The Sleep Sense Program: Proven Strategies For Teaching Your Child To Sleep Through The Night*, p. 10.

9. Safe to Sleep. (nd). Frequently asked questions (FAQs) about SIDS and safe infant sleep. Retrieved from https://safetosleep.nichd.nih.gov/safesleepbasics/faq.

10. Parker-Pope, T. (2008). Fan in baby's room lowers SIDS risk. *The New York Times*. Retrieved from https://well.blogs.nytimes.com/2008/10/06/embargo-fan-in-babys-room-lowers-sids-risk/.

CHAPTER 3: WEEK ONE

1. Unicef. (n.d.). Skin-to-skin contact. Retrieved from https://www.unicef.org.uk/babyfriendly/baby-friendly-resources/implementing-standards-resources/skin-to-skin-contact/.

2. Ezzo, G. & Bucknam, R. (2006). *On Becoming Babywise: Giving Your Infant the Gift of Nighttime Sleep (4ᵗʰ edition)*, p. 76.

3. Greenfield, P. & Fields, L. (2018). Parents. 16 things you didn't know about breastfeeding. Retrieved from https://www.parents.com/baby/breastfeeding/10-things-you-didnt-know-about-breastfeeding/

CHAPTER 4: WEEK TWO
   1. Ezzo, G. & Bucknam, R. (2006). *On Becoming Babywise: Giving Your Infant the Gift of Nighttime Sleep (4th edition)*, p. 112.
   2. The American Academy of Pediatrics. (2016). American Academy of Pediatrics announces new recommendations for children's media use. https://www.aap.org/en-us/about-the-aap/aap-press-room/Pages/American-Academy-of-Pediatrics-Announces-New-Recommendations-for-Childrens-Media-Use.aspx
   3. Weissbluth, M. (2015). *Healthy Sleep Habits, Happy Child (Fourth edition)*, p. 453.
   4. Ezzo, G. & Bucknam, R. (2006). *On Becoming Babywise: Giving Your Infant the Gift of Nighttime Sleep (4th edition)*, p. 130.
   5. Ezzo, G. & Bucknam, R. (2006). *On Becoming Babywise: Giving Your Infant the Gift of Nighttime Sleep (4th edition)*, p. 49.
   6. Mayo Clinic. (2019). Spitting up in babies: What's normal, what's not. Retrieved from https://www.mayoclinic.org/healthy-lifestyle/infant-and-toddler-health/in-depth/healthy-baby/art-20044329

CHAPTER 5: WEEK THREE
   1. Weissbluth, M. (2015). *Healthy Sleep Habits, Happy Child (Fourth edition)*, p. 133.
   2. Karp, H. (2015). *The Happiest Baby on the Block: The New Way to Calm Crying and Help Your Newborn Baby Sleep Longer*. Retrieved from

https://www.happiestbaby.com/blogs/baby/the-5-s-s-for-soothing-babies

CHAPTER 7: NORMAL DEVELOPMENT: 1 MONTH
1. Ezzo, G. & Bucknam, R. (2006). *On Becoming Babywise: Giving Your Infant the Gift of Nighttime Sleep (4ᵗʰ edition),* p. 112.
2. Bright Futures Parent Handout: 1 Month Visit. Retrieved from Bright Futures (AAP); www.brightfutures.aap.org
3. Ezzo, G. & Bucknam, R. (2006). *On Becoming Babywise: Giving Your Infant the Gift of Nighttime Sleep (4ᵗʰ edition),* p. 92-93.

CHAPTER 8: WEEK FIVE
1. Weissbluth, M. (2015). *Healthy Sleep Habits, Happy Child (Fourth edition),* p. 132.
2. The American Academy of Pediatrics. (2016). SIDS and other sleep-related infant deaths: updated 2016 recommendations for a safe infant sleeping environment. Retrieved from: https://pediatrics.aappublications.org/content/138/5/e201 62938
3. The American Academy of Pediatrics. (2016). SIDS and other sleep-related infant deaths: updated 2016 recommendations for a safe infant sleeping environment. Retrieved from: https://pediatrics.aappublications.org/content/138/5/e201 62938

CHAPTER 9: WEEK SIX
1. Ezzo, G. & Bucknam, R. (2006). *On Becoming Babywise: Giving Your Infant the Gift of Nighttime Sleep (4ᵗʰ edition),* p. 114.

2. Weissbluth, M. (2015). *Healthy Sleep Habits, Happy Child (Fourth edition)*, p. 203.

CHAPTER 11: WEEK EIGHT
1. The American Academy of Pediatrics. (2017). Swaddling: Is it safe? Retrieved from https://www.healthychildren.org/English/ages-stages/baby/diapers-clothing/Pages/Swaddling-Is-it-Safe.aspx

CHAPTER 12: NORMAL DEVELOPMENT: 2 MONTHS
1. Bright Futures Parent Handout: 2 Month Visit. Retrieved from Bright Futures (AAP); www.brightfutures.aap.org

CHAPTER 14: THREE TO FIVE MONTHS
1. Obleman, D. (2007). *The Sleep Sense Program: Proven Strategies For Teaching Your Child To Sleep Through The Night*, p. 71-72.
2. Essential Baby. (2008). Early bedtime means better sleep. Retrieved from http://www.essentialbaby.com.au/baby/baby-sleep/early-bedtime-means-better-sleep-20080506-2bip
3. Weissbluth, M. (2015). *Healthy Sleep Habits, Happy Child (Fourth edition)*, p. 30.

CHAPTER 15: NORMAL DEVELOPMENT: 6 MONTHS
1. Bright Futures Parent Handout: 6 Month Visit. Retrieved from Bright Futures (AAP); www.brightfutures.aap.org

CHAPTER 16: SIX TO NINE MONTHS
1. The American Academy of Pediatrics. (2013). Early introduction of allergenic foods may prevent food

allergy in children. Retrieved from
https://www.aappublications.org/

CHAPTER 17: NORMAL DEVELOPMENT: 9 MONTHS
1. Bright Futures Parent Handout: 9 Month Visit. Retrieved from Bright Futures (AAP); www.brightfutures.aap.org

CHAPTER 19: NORMAL DEVELOPMENT: 12 MONTHS
1. Bright Futures Parent Handout: 12 Month Visit. Retrieved from Bright Futures (AAP); www.brightfutures.aap.org

23

ABOUT THE AUTHOR

TAYLOR FONTENOT is a Registered Nurse, mom to three, cancer survivor, Georgia native, and the original Baby Sleep Boss. She is most known for her sense of adventure and her tendency to cry happy tears with wildlife sightings.

Taylor and her husband, Michael, live in Fort Collins, Colorado. They spent the first stint of their marriage traveling the world and visiting over 25 countries together, but they both agree that the real adventure began with parenthood in 2014. They now have three sons – Kepler, Crew, and Lincoln – and enjoy family road trips, hiking, camping, and traveling around their beautiful state and beyond.

Since becoming a mom, Taylor has grown passionate about guiding "the next generation" of parents through the highs and lows of their baby's first year. Check here for more:

Website: www.thebabysleepboss.com
Instagram: taylorbfontenot